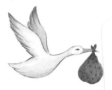

D0878453

Praise for NATURAL HOSPITAL BIRTH

"Cynthia Gabriel's book is of paramount importance for those women who choose a hospital birth and who would like to minimize disturbance and interference with normal physiological labor and birth. She offers women a vast array of carefully crafted, thoughtful, and practical suggestions that rise from her rich experiences as a mother, doula, therapist, and anthropologist."

—MARY SHARPE, PH.D., M.ED., REGISTERED MIDWIFE

"All deliveries are wonderful, but a natural birth in a hospital is an amazing experience for all involved. As an obstetrician, I meet many couples who would like both a natural birth and the safeguards of the hospital setting. This book helps parents-to-be raise their awareness and expand their options about possibilities, and it provides concrete steps for working with their providers to achieve the goal of a natural birth in a hospital."

—FRANK J. ANDERSON, M.D., M.P.P., UNIVERSITY OF MICHIGAN

"Written with clarity, sensitivity, and thoroughness, *Natural Hospital Birth* offers the information and encouragement that can make a critical difference for new parents and their babies. This is essential reading, not just for those planning a hospital birth, but also for those planning a home birth, so they can be prepared for all eventualities. *Natural Hospital Birth* belongs in every midwife's library."

—JAN HUNT, DIRECTOR OF THE NATIONAL CHILD PROJECT AND AUTHOR OF
THE NATURAL CHILD: PARENTING FROM THE HEART AND A GIFT FOR BABY

"Many women desire natural birth, but few women in the United States experience it. Each birth represents an opportunity for growth and empowerment, but too often women feel disappointed afterward, as though they have failed or been failed, or even been traumatized by their experience . . . As a doula, Cynthia Gabriel is uniquely positioned to understand what works and what does not work in hospitals. She knows the many tried-and-true techniques for helping women cope with the challenges of labor . . . and tells the truth about what it takes to have a natural birth in a hospital."

—JULIA SENG, PH.D., R.N., CERTIFIED NURSE-MIDWIFE, CO-AUTHOR OF
***SURVIVOR MOMS*, AND RESEARCH ASSOCIATE PROFESSOR AT THE UNIVERSITY OF MICHIGAN INSTITUTE FOR RESEARCH ON WOMEN AND GENDER**

"A beautiful and practical guide to normal birth in the hospital, *Natural Hospital Birth* is the perfect resource for pregnant women, doulas, and midwives who value the normalcy of birth and who feel it should be a woman's right in any setting. In clear terms, Cynthia Gabriel empowers women with the information they need to advocate and plan for a natural birth."

—ERIN GRAHAM, MASSAGE THERAPIST, DOULA, AND INTERIM DIRECTOR OF BIRTH FOCUS

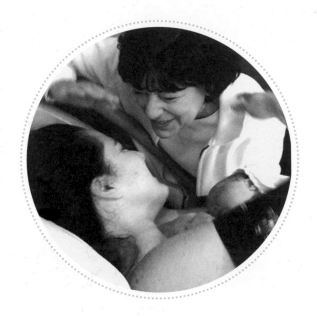

For Jamie Muchmaker,

*the most natural, inspiring mother I have ever met,
and for my Aunt Marietta*

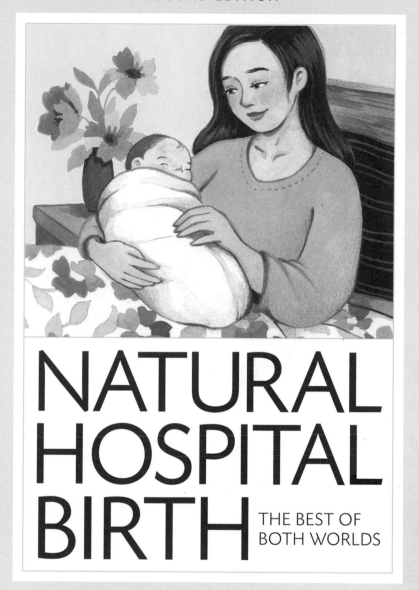

NATURAL HOSPITAL BIRTH

THE BEST OF BOTH WORLDS

CYNTHIA GABRIEL

Foreword by Timothy R. B. Johnson, M.D.,
OB-GYN, University of Michigan

HARVARD COMMON PRESS

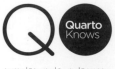

Brimming with creative inspiration, how-to projects, and useful information to enrich your everyday life, Quarto Knows is a favorite destination for those pursuing their interests and passions. Visit our site and dig deeper with our books into your area of interest: Quarto Creates, Quarto Cooks, Quarto Homes, Quarto Lives, Quarto Drives, Quarto Explores, Quarto Gifts, or Quarto Kids.

First Published in 2018 by The Harvard Common Press, an imprint of The Quarto Group, 100 Cummings Center, Suite 265-D, Beverly, MA 01915, USA.
T (978) 282-9590 F (978) 283-2742 QuartoKnows.com

The Harvard Common Press titles are also available at discount for retail, wholesale, promotional, and bulk purchase. For details, contact the Special Sales Manager by email at specialsales@quarto.com or by mail at The Quarto Group, Attn: Special Sales Manager, 401 Second Avenue North, Suite 310, Minneapolis, MN 55401, USA.

22 21 20 19 18   1 2 3 4 5

ISBN: 978-1-55832-917-1

Originally found under the following Library of Congress Cataloging-in-Publication Data
Gabriel, Cynthia.
  Natural hospital birth : the best of both worlds / Cynthia Gabriel ; foreword by Timothy R. B. Johnson.
      p. cm.
  Includes bibliographical references and index.
  ISBN 978-1-55832-718-4 (pbk. : alk. paper)
  1. Natural childbirth--Popular works. I. Title.
  RG661.G33 2011
  618.4'5--dc22
                                        2010019882

Cover design by Laura H. Couallier, Laura Herrmann Design
Cover illustration by Susie So
Interior design by Laura H. Couallier, Laura Herrmann Design
Layout: *tabula rasa* graphic design
Illustrations by Keleigh Lee

Printed in China

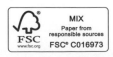

Contents

Foreword

EVERYTHING GOES IN CYCLES IN MEDICINE and in health care, just as in life. Cynthia Gabriel's new book comes at a fortuitous "sweet spot," when obstetric birth practices in the United States are again changing. As I write this, the American College of Obstetricians and Gynecologists is liberalizing its statement on vaginal birth after cesarean delivery (VBAC) with the hope of expanding the use of VBAC, especially in smaller and rural hospitals, where it has been largely abandoned.

With fathers now in attendance in operating rooms and extended families at vaginal births, and with increasing choices for pain relief and support persons, *Natural Hospital Birth* will allow for improved collaboration and negotiation around these choices. It will be very useful not only to birthing women but also to physicians, nurse-midwives, nurses, health policy makers, and hospital administrators. The twenty-first century is a time for collaboration: Midwives, family physicians, obstetric anesthesiologists, labor nurses, obstetrician-gynecologists, and often high-risk obstetricians and neonatologists are collaborating in a much more constructive way than ever before, but they are doing so in an increasingly medicalized environment. This is the environment where Cynthia Gabriel focuses the lens for her book.

Pregnant women seem to be turning away from childbirth education and turning toward epidural anesthesia. "I learned everything I need from a video," some say, whether it was a reality TV show or a professionally prepared educational video. Patients are getting more information than ever before, in many new ways, but how are they processing the information? How are they using it to negotiate the care they want? It is time once again for women to educate themselves, as they did in the 1960s and 1970s, with books like *Our Bodies, Ourselves*. In fact, the Boston Women's Health Book Collective has recently published *Our Bodies, Ourselves: Pregnancy and Birth*, which provides just the kind of detailed factual information that pregnant (or, better yet, soon-to-be pregnant) women need. *Natural Hospital Birth* will be an invaluable supplement for women who want to put such factual knowledge about childbirth into use. Cynthia Gabriel takes a balanced view as she clarifies not only the medical evidence but also the biases that lead practitioners, family physicians, obstetricians, and nurse-midwives to do the things that they do. Unquestionably, these things will change. Readers can use this book to bring about constructive, positive changes that will improve women's birth experiences while making sure that safety is paramount.

Nature often presents unexpected challenges, and these need to be anticipated and accepted. For those women who select the relative safety of a modern hospital as one way to handle the unexpected, reduce risks, and increase access to resources when the unexpected happens, Cynthia Gabriel gives good advice. I always try to remember and teach that childbirth is a natural process that with little or no intervention normally turns out well. But nature does not assure a perfect or even a good outcome. Unfortunately, in too many low-income countries today, women die in childbirth. We are lucky in the United States that birth has become so safe that we can now focus on the quality of the birth experience. (Our childbirth movement has provided a lesson for developing countries: It is a benefit—in fact, a right—for every laboring woman to have a support person, if not a support network, during pregnancy, in labor and delivery, and during the postpartum period. Having birth is safer when you're surrounded by people you can trust who can look out for and advocate for your interests.)

Particularly rich is Cynthia Gabriel's chapter on birth plans. I ask all my pregnant patients at least to think through, and preferably to write out, a birth plan. Even in the most conservative and unaccommodating hospitals, laboring mothers have many potential advocates. These advocates, most often labor nurses but occasionally birth educators, ombudspersons, social workers, lactation consultants, pain nurses or nurse anesthetists, doulas, and others, can be better advocates if they have a clear idea of a patient's wishes. There is no better roadmap for advocates to follow than a birth plan that is clearly written and succinct (be careful—no one will finish reading a fifteen-page document). In fact, a good birth plan will serve as an invaluable roadmap for any labor nurse, anesthesiologist, or other care provider a patient comes in contact with, even in the ideal birth environment.

Natural Hospital Birth is, to my knowledge, the first detailed book on pregnancy and labor that is written by a doula—and a doula with a developed anthropologic perspective. Like any good ethnographer, Cynthia Gabriel includes plenty of stories in her book. These birth narratives make the material very accessible. After all, any labor anywhere could be the subject of an engrossing soap opera or reality TV show.

Pregnancy, childbirth, and new parenthood are too anticipated, too personal, and too important not to deserve careful preparation, not just for their immediate and long-term effects on the physical health of a woman and her infant but for their long-term effects on the mother's mental health and self-confidence and the family's dynamics. Professionally written print and electronic media, childbirth classes, and now *Natural Hospital Birth* are the kinds of resources that empower birthing women. I will add this book to the list of recommended resources I give to all my patients.

—Timothy R. B. Johnson
Chair of the Department of Obstetrics and Gynecology
Professor of Women's Studies
University of Michigan

Acknowledgments

I HAVE LEARNED FROM BIRTH WORK TO APPRECIATE the women who have gone before me: my mother, Maura Smith Gabriel, and my grandmothers, Laura Tolman Smith and Matilda Bernt Gabriel. Thank you to all the mothers who shared their stories. I hope I have done them justice.

I have been blessed on my pathway to writing this book with the companionship and guidance of more than my share of angels. Without the people I thank here, I know this book would never have been born.

I owe my appreciation and understanding of natural birth to a long list of people, some of whom I can mention here. First is Nancy Chen, Ph.D. In a medical anthropology course at the University of California, Santa Cruz, she told a personal, empowering story about giving birth. That led me to a life-altering doula training class with Ann Fuller and a midwifery class with Elizabeth Davis. Ann and Elizabeth said many wise words, but what I remember most from Ann is the admonition that "no birth you attend is yours" and Elizabeth's advice to embrace fear at birth. Thank you to Elizabeth Davis, also, for commenting on and improving several chapters. Elvira Zakublovskaya, obstetrician-gynecologist and homebirth midwife in Nizhni Novgorod, Russia, graciously shared her life with me in 2000. I am deeply grateful to Molly Rybak for my experience as a midwifery student on the Russian Birth Project (RBP). While apprenticing at the RBP, I also learned from Kristina Chamberlain and Bonnie Martin, who are now wonderful midwives.

I could never have written this book if I had not been supported by so much love at my own children's births. I am so grateful to my midwives: Joan Bryson, Linda Moscovitch, Chris Sternberg, Mary Sharpe, and Mickey Sperlich. Joan supported me through the fears and insecurities of my first pregnancy and birth, never doubting that I would have a beautiful birth experience. Linda calmly handled my second pregnancy (including two external versions), Chris brilliantly told me to "put your leg up in the air and push!" when my son's shoulders got stuck, and Mary gently called me back to Earth when I felt like I was floating away after his whirlwind entry. This last birth with Mickey taught me many lessons that I will mine for many years. I am so appreciative of Mickey for her wisdom, humor, friendship, and collaborative spirit. The full moon did not induce my labor the night she showed it to me, but I still believe that Mickey's midwifery is magic.

Theresa Gabriel, Amy Tatko, Tracey Reid, Lavetta Griffin, Charlie Clayton, Anna Verriest, Kary Young, Melissa Palma, Pam Maturo, Kendra Theriot, Patrick Soule, Jillean McCommons, Valerie Taylor, Amy Advey, Erin Reid, Barbara Roberston, Kate Stroud, Keleigh Lee, and many, many others supported me with great love (including baking brownies while I was in labor, tattooing my belly, and taking care of my other children) as a birthing woman. Melissa and Kary, there is much in my life that wouldn't have happened without you. The AIDS LifeCycle (a 545-mile [877 km] fundraising bike ride down the California coast), a book, and a baby: You were there for it all.

As a doula, I acknowledge four mothers whose experiences have profoundly shaped me. I feel honored to have attended them in labor: Amy Allington, Amy Tatko, Jamie Muchmaker, and my sister, Debi Fairman. Your children, Misha, Sadie, Tessa, and Katelyn, hold special places in my heart. Dave and Ritu were too far away to invite me to their birth in India, but I thank them for the chance to first set down in writing a guide for "how to get a natural birth in a hospital."

As an extrovert, I wish I could have talked my book into existence. Instead, I found I had to do a lot of solitary writing. My writing coach, Dave Storer, and writing group helped me stay the course. Dave, LeAnn Keenan, and Zoe Clarkwest read a remarkable number of drafts with enthusiasm. Thank you for all your advice, hand-holding, chocolate, and coffee. You made this book a celebration. Naomi Wolf and Wende Jager-Hyman at the Woodhull Institute generously helped find the "hook" of this book. Leah Mundell, Sasha Welland, and Mae Lee, my companions at the University of California, Santa Cruz, offered helpful advice on early drafts and encouragement through graduate school and fieldwork. Brenda Gabriel has offered her editing genius on occasions too numerous to count.

Julia Seng, Ph.D., C.N.M., gave me the opportunity to work on her project "Stress and the Childbearing Year" at the University of Michigan. I can't imagine life in Ann Arbor without her support of me as a person and as a scholar. Julia's expert eyes helped improve a final draft of this book. Frank Anderson, M.D., M.P.H., also gave generously of his time to read several chapters and help me understand a physician's point of view.

There would be no book on the shelves if it weren't for Kate Epstein, my talented agent. When I first envisioned this book, I told my writing group that I hoped to find an agent who felt passionate about the message of this book. I feel blessed that my wish came true. She guided me to The Harvard Common Press and editor Linda Ziedrich. Linda's precision with language amazes me.

Finally, I would like to acknowledge and thank from the deepest parts of my heart the people who have not only supported my lifelong journey but are currently walking with me: my family and closest friends.

My sisters, Debi, Brenda, Cheri, and Theresa, have supported me in ways that only sisters can. My parents-in-law, Wulf and Renate Paulick, have exhibited real interest in this book from its conception. Renate keeps me up-to-date with anything birth-related that makes it into the news.

Maria Aliberti and Amy Tatko are two sisters I didn't grow up with, but that life provided me. Maria is waiting for her first child to arrive. Auntie Cynthia is eager for the arrival and the many hours of birth storytelling to follow! Maria's interest in all things related to nature, including natural birth, inspires me. Amy Tatko flew from California to New York to be at my daughter's birth and then invited me to make the reverse journey a year later for her daughter's birth. We started out friends because we both loved Russia, but we have shared much more than that in the years between giggly girlhood and natural mamahood. Amy is an amazing writer, and I have benefited enormously from her editing and writing guidance. I thank Amy for taking my interest in birth to heart when it was first developing. I also send her approximately three thousand semicolons that, if it weren't for Amy, would have made it into this book.

Felix, thank you for being my true partner and for being the father I always hoped to find for my children. Thank you for all the hours—turned into years—that you have supported this book, by talking about it, by ignoring the piles of papers all over our house, and by giving me child-free hours to work. I often needed to borrow your confidence to keep going. Your faith in me is a gift.

While birthing this book, I also birthed our third child, Anju. Sylvia, Calvin, and Anju are the reason that giving birth is so full of joy and meaning for me. I am astonished by the people they are becoming, and I am so grateful that they picked me to be their mother.

As I revise this book in 2017, I am grateful for so many people who are vital to my continued development as a birth researcher and doula, including all these people and many more: Jessica English, Heather Boyd, Connie Bonnie Perkins, Patrice Bobier, Joanne Motino Bailey, Lesley Everest, Amanda Howell, Stacia Proefrock, Cynthia Jackson, Jessica Walker, Jennifer D'Jamoos, and Kelly Hill Aronoff. You have each contributed to the revision of this book, though you may not even know it. Jessica English, editor extraordinaire, found many important places that needed revision. Some of you sent me articles or answered questions; others just kept me informed and up-to-date through your beautiful Facebook presence. Lesley Everest graciously invited me into MotherWit world as a doula trainer. I am especially grateful to the constant support and friendship of my Tree Town Doula compatriots: Catherine Fischer, Toni Aucker, Martha Baum, Gillian Lee, and Ana Fernandez.

Introduction

WHEN I SET OUT TO WRITE THIS BOOK, I thought my perspective as a birthing mother was my most important resource. Certainly, my own experiences giving birth (one cesarean section after a wonderful natural labor, and two all-natural vaginal births) color my ideas about birth. But as I worked, I realized that my most valuable resources are my experience as a doula supporting women in hospital birth and the trust in birth that I developed as an anthropologist.

The point of view of a doula is distinct from that of an obstetrician or midwife. Doulas notice different things about birth than medical care providers do.

When I read a book about natural birth authored by a physician, I realized that certain aspects of the hospital experience are invisible to her. She is never in the room when a birthing woman has to negotiate a medical procedure with a nurse. Since this physician is supportive of natural birth, she has not observed women fighting for a natural birth with an unsupportive caregiver. She does not drive to a family's home to support early labor and help a woman know the right time to go to the hospital. Physicians do not often hold a client's hand for two hours as she cries about a previous miscarriage while she is in the midst of labor.

So, although it is true that obstetricians know a lot about birth that doulas do not know, it is also true that doulas know a lot about birth that obstetricians do not know.

My experience as an anthropologist also gives me a unique window onto hospital birth. I understand birth from an evolutionary and cross-cultural perspective. Whereas doctors attend years of medical school to understand the physiology of our bodily processes, I attended years of graduate school to understand the culture and meaning of our bodily processes. In particular, my research into Russian birth gives me a comparative understanding of our own hospital practices. Anthropologists know that seeing anything—a family, a church, or a birth—in another culture makes it possible to see details of our own experience that were previously imperceptible.

What I brought back with me from a year of studying birth in Russia was an unshakable faith that natural birth can occur in the hospital setting. Of sixty-six births that I witnessed, only one was medicated. In North America, witnessing two natural hospital births in a row is rare. Most American doctors and midwives do not have the opportunity to witness natural hospital birth over and over again.

Why do American women so seldom experience natural hospital birth? Why can't American women endure the pain of labor? While many birth researchers blame doctors and a century of medicalized childbirth, I have a different idea. I answer this question as an anthropologist. Two aspects of our culture seem particularly vital. The first is structural. We all live with constraints imposed on us by the structures of our health-care system, the insurance business, and laws regarding liability. (Obstetricians are the most-sued doctors in the United States. An average obstetrician is sued three times in a career and each suit can last four to five years. Russian doctors and midwives are paid by the government; Russia has virtually no insurance companies; and none of the Russian doctors whom I interviewed had ever been sued by a patient.) The second aspect is related to our cultural values. Simply put, our culture does not honor birth pain.

Here in the United States and Canada, our culture doesn't teach us that birth pain leads to something valuable. Our society fails to recognize the merit of most pain, not just birth pain, and we go to great lengths to avoid unpleasant feelings. So many North American women have experienced the pain of labor, and then an epidural, that our collective memory about birth is now full of hurt but is missing the feelings of ecstasy and success that natural birth provides. A few women compare the feeling of birth to orgasm. Though this is not how most women describe it, I think the comparison to an intense, positive feeling of release after an extensive buildup makes sense. In Russia, by contrast, suffering is considered an admirable pathway to becoming a better person. Russians from all walks of life can speak eloquently about positive transformation through pain. Russia is not unique. Most other cultures in the world provide a lifelong message to girls and women that the physical labor of birth is not just valuable, it is heroic. To embrace the pain of labor, we must reclaim its value.

I hope that *Natural Hospital Birth: The Best of Both Worlds* will help women and their care providers appreciate the value of natural birth in their lives. We cannot easily change the insurance or legal systems by ourselves, but we can, each of us, reflect on the meaning of pain in our lives and make new decisions about what we will value and enjoy. Yes, we can even enjoy giving birth.

When I talk with a woman who is nervous about giving birth, who is intimidated by stories of complications, and who believes that everyone needs drugs to get through labor, I do not tell her about medical studies, facts and figures, or side effects of drugs. I do not talk about what labor feels like. Instead, I tell her this one truth that matters more than any of those facts: I love giving birth.

I love it. I enjoy it. I would happily do it many more times in my lifetime if I could. My three children's births could not have been more different from one another. My experiences of labor were intense. I felt great pain (not just "surges" or "sensations," as some describe contractions). I do not love giving birth because it is easy or pain-free.

I love birth because when my body is bringing forth new life I feel vibrant, important, and certain that the work I am doing is worthwhile. I learn the value of giving up control and accepting life as it is. Once, this has even meant accepting that my baby's birth was not going to happen the way I wanted.

The best Russian births and the best American births, the best home-births and the best hospital births, have one thing in common: a sense among all persons present that this birth is sacred. This attitude, I have come to believe, is far more important than the room in which a woman gives birth.

I hope that this book will help you to overcome our culture's messages and find your own power and strength as a birthing woman. No one can predict the physical aspects of your labor, but I have learned that if you bring all of yourself—your emotions, your intellect, your body, and your spirit—to your baby's birth, you will be rewarded. I wish for you what I have received in my life: the ability to look back on giving birth with peace and joy.

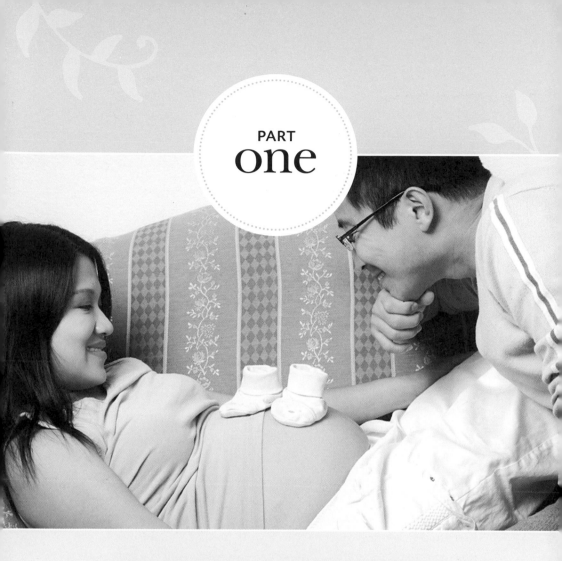

PART
one

PREPARING FOR YOUR BABY'S BIRTH

CHAPTER 1

YOU CAN DO IT

S O YOU WANT A NATURAL BIRTH.

And, by choice or by circumstance, you will give birth in a hospital. You can do it!

You will be fighting against the odds, yet a natural birth in the hospital is possible. It is feasible. Your hope is very realistic.

In these pages, you will meet women who achieved natural births in hospitals all over North America, as well as their partners and their loved ones. Their stories are inspiring and can teach you what it takes to give birth naturally.

If you are like the majority of women in North America, you are interested in letting your body follow its natural course in labor the same way that it has followed its natural course during your pregnancy. You are curious, apprehensive, or perhaps even scared about facing labor pain. You may believe that having access to the high-tech specialists and equipment of a hospital will put your mind at ease. But you hope that high-tech interventions will be saved for a serious emergency, when they are absolutely necessary.

Perhaps you have always known that you will give birth in a hospital. Or perhaps you have investigated giving birth at home or in a birth center. Yet your thoughts or research have led you to decide that these options are not right for you. Many women cannot explain why, but they know that they feel safest giving birth in a hospital. Other women would be interested in out-of-hospital options, but those options are not available or affordable where they live. And still other women find themselves in a "high-risk" category that makes out-of-hospital birth medically inadvisable.

The bottom line is that you desire a natural birth and you feel safest giving birth in a hospital. Setting the intention to achieve a natural hospital birth is a wonderful first step. Women merit the right to choose hospital birth without having to sacrifice the body's natural process. There is no good reason that pregnant women in North America should not be able to have what they most deeply desire. Natural birth in hospitals is possible.

What it requires is taking responsibility and consciously preparing for your birth experience. Yes, you must trust many people around you to do their part. Yet, ultimately, this labor is yours. Once an egg and sperm have met and implanted in your body, no one else can turn them into a human being except you. You, and no one else, are responsible for birthing this baby.

This concept may sound weighty, yet it is also freeing. Your partner, your mother, your best friend, and your doctor have opinions about how you should give birth. If you asked me or any stranger on the street, we would probably have an opinion about how you should give birth. But none of us have to live in your body, in your mind, in your emotions, with your decisions. You do.

In a hospital, you will be surrounded by authority figures who probably have far more knowledge than you of fetal heartbeats and blood vessels in an umbilical cord. These authority figures have expertise and skills. They also have intuition and personal histories and unique personalities. You get all of these when you choose a doctor or midwife and a hospital.

You are also surrounded by protocols—lists of "best practices" that the hospital puts out as its internal "laws." Protocols are strong guidelines for hospital staff and physicians. Though midwives and doctors can make decisions that are outside of protocol, they are usually reluctant to do so because this would increase their risk of a liability suit. Yet protocols vary greatly. One hospital might sanction women going twenty-four hours without intervention after their waters break, while another hospital might endorse a shorter time of only twelve hours. One hospital may ask women not to eat or drink during a natural labor; another hospital may encourage women to nourish themselves at will.

You get to decide how much power to give these authority figures and protocols. Though they can be intimidating and even coercive, ultimately, no doctor can do anything to you without your consent. If you have experienced interventions in a previous birth, you already know how difficult it can be to maintain your confidence when a complication arises. However, you do have power. Doctors have authoritative knowledge. But so do you. Your body possesses wisdom and knowledge that no clinician could ever match.

One example illustrates this. Fetal monitors are routinely used for most hospital births in North America. Belts around the woman's belly measure the fetal heartbeat and the frequency of the woman's contractions. A computer screen displays this information. The monitor appears to display the intensity of contractions, but in fact, external monitors cannot measure the intensity of contractions—only duration and frequency. At the first hospital birth I ever attended, I was struck by how the nurses and the grandmother-to-be watched the computer screen rather than the face of t   he laboring woman, Rachel. When Rachel said that a contraction was "the worst one yet" her mother replied, "No, it wasn't. The one before went much higher." Our bodies know how to measure pain better than a machine does.

Situations can arise in which your desire for a natural birth and your body's wisdom might seem to be at odds with your caregiver's advice or hospital protocol. Experiencing this tension can be scary. Indeed, fear is the most common reaction to this situation. Many natural-birth advocates are deeply afraid of obstetrical practices. This apprehension can lead to an unfortunate situation in which a woman considers her care providers to be opponents instead of trusted allies.

As I will discuss in a later chapter, fear has dire consequences for birth. If a woman's subconscious thinks there is an enemy in the room, it will shut down labor. It is vital that you see your caregiver as a member of your team, someone who is on your side. I believe it is possible to do this even when you disagree with your caregiver.

How do you do this? First, you must create a vision of birth for yourself. Then, you must communicate, to everyone with whom you interact, your commitment and desire to give birth naturally. In my experience as a doula, I have watched some tough-minded nurses and dogmatic doctors—the ones who normally bring out all the techno-wizardry at the slightest provocation—melt under the spell of a woman's commitment to natural birth. When care providers believe that a woman is committed—that she is fully informed, fully prepared, and genuinely speaking from her heart—they may walk through fire to help her get the birth experience that she desires. I will discuss how to create this team atmosphere in much greater detail later.

Some medical caregivers, especially labor-and-delivery nurses, can and do offer the trust and commitment that allow a woman to experience natural birth. I interviewed a woman in Toronto who remembers how her nurse coached her through each contraction and kept telling her she was doing wonderfully. Even though this woman hadn't planned to do so, she ended up giving birth naturally. Most of the time, however, the key factor is the commitment of the birthing woman.

You may have hoped that if you shopped carefully for your care provider, you would be able to just go along with whatever this practitioner suggests. In fact, this is the tack most women take and many pregnancy books support. Though many authors advocate learning about your options, few help you evaluate the suggestions your care provider may give you. This book aims to give you the tools you need to use the recommendations of your care provider wisely and in ways that work best for you.

What Is a Natural Birth?

Natural birth is defined differently by different people. Natural birth can refer to any of the following, alone or in combination:

• Vaginal birth, with or without the use of pharmaceutical drugs

• Birth without pain-relieving drugs

• Birth without any drugs whatsoever

- Birth with only select interventions allowed, according to the mother's birth plan

- Birth with the fewest interventions possible to support the health of the mother and baby

In this book, natural birth means the most instinctive, self-directed, intervention-free birth possible.

Some birth experts prefer the term *physiologic birth*, which the American College of Nurse-Midwives describes as birth "that is powered by the innate human capacity of the woman and fetus." Although I, too, like the precision of *physiologic birth*, I do not think it is going to become a household term anytime soon. I find the phrase *physiologic birth* most useful when I am speaking with medically trained professionals, not when I am working with pregnant women. I have chosen to retain the phrase *natural birth* for this book because it is the way we tend to speak in everyday conversation.

Every birth is unique. Just as each one of us is a unique person, so too are our beginnings in this world. Though we may be able to group together some births as "more natural" and others as "more interventionist," each birth is the culmination of an absolutely unrepeatable pregnancy. It represents a physical, emotional, and spiritual relationship between a mother and baby, as well as a unique set of circumstances. What is natural for one woman and one baby may seem artificial to another.

The acceptable level of intervention varies across a spectrum of possibilities. In the end, there is no such thing as a birth free from human intervention. We are among a select group of mammals, which include dolphins and elephants, who prefer to give birth in the company of others. Even that company is an intervention.

For the majority of women, a natural birth means giving birth spontaneously (without induction), at one's own pace (without drugs to increase the speed), and under one's own power (without anesthetics). Most women alive today would be able to give birth safely without any medical support. For very few babies and even fewer women, medical intervention is necessary during the birth process. For these women, natural birth means the most natural birth possible. When intervention is unavoidable, the task is to identify the minimum level of intervention necessary.

A woman's commitment to natural birth does not end because she faces an emergency complication. It simply changes. Her agreement to one intervention does not necessarily mean that she welcomes others. Unfortunately, when one medical intervention is performed, others become statistically more likely. This proven effect is known as the Cascade.

The stories of two women, Sam and Joanna, are illustrative. Both women were absolutely committed to natural birth. In both cases, medical problems led them to accept interventions, but they worked hard to prevent these interventions from medicalizing the rest of their experience.

Sam agreed to have prophylactic antibiotics during labor because she had tested positive for group B strep.* She arranged to have the antibiotics administered at two separate times. After each administration, her midwives disconnected the intravenous line (IV) so that she could move freely during labor. Many practitioners leave women attached to the IV after the first dose of antibiotics to make it easier to administer subsequent doses, but Sam didn't want to be attached to an IV in active labor. Her energetic labor, in and out of a birth tub, would certainly have been hindered by an IV pole. A saline lock (also called a hep lock, saline or hep trap, an IV port, or, if you live in Colorado, a "buff cap"), which keeps the vein open for subsequent doses of antibiotics, was a practical compromise that allowed her free movement in labor.

Even in circumstances that preclude physiologic birth, a woman can still insist on a minimum of intervention. Joanna, a chiropractor by profession, gave birth by cesarean section because at nine months her baby was positioned foot-first (instead of head- or bottom-first, either of which would allow a vaginal delivery). Joanna tried special chiropractic maneuvers and external version (an attempt to turn a baby to a better position by pressing on the mother's abdomen), to no avail. She insisted on holding her baby immediately after birth, while she was on the operating table. She was also adamant about sharing a bed with her infant in the hospital.

---

* Group B strep is a vaginal bacterium that is found in about 20 percent of healthy women. Administering antibiotics is standard protocol in North America to help the tiny percentage of babies who would otherwise be harmed by group B strep during birth. In most of the world, women are not tested for group B strep and therefore are not treated for it.

You have many decisions to make—some that you can make ahead of time, and others that you may have to make on the spot—when choosing what intervention is acceptable to you. As you develop your birth plan, it will become easier to make these choices because you will become increasingly conscious of the pattern of reasoning you are following.

Take a moment to reflect and write about what natural birth means to you. There are probably images or words that flash in your mind whenever you hear the word *birth*. Pay attention to these. Think about them and what they might mean to you. Why do you desire a natural birth?

You may be concerned about health, both yours and the baby's. You may want to avoid unnecessary chemicals in your body or a needle in your spine. You may want to know that your baby will have the best shot at breathing well and bonding with you right after birth. You are probably trying to decrease your odds of having a cesarean section.

A desire to avoid a cesarean is understandable because the experience of a C-section can be traumatic and dangerous. The list of complications from C-sections is daunting: More mothers die from the surgery than from giving birth vaginally; mothers who have C-sections can experience serious complications in future pregnancies; babies born by C-section have more trouble breathing right away and also in the long term, and they have more trouble breastfeeding than do babies born vaginally. Most mothers who give birth surgically have epidurals or spinal anesthesia, and they therefore also experience the risks associated with epidurals, including a "spinal headache" and nerve damage. In addition, it is much harder to take care of a newborn while trying to recover from major surgery.

But you may also be motivated by something beyond health statistics. I have heard proponents of anesthetized birth say, "There's no medal for birthing naturally." For many women, though, natural birth brings the greatest reward that any life experience can provide—a sense of joy, achievement, and satisfaction. Through this physical, mental, and emotional challenge, you will know yourself and your body more deeply than you ever could otherwise. You will recognize your own physical, mental, and emotional strength. Or, as Lesley Everest, a doula trainer in Montreal, puts it so eloquently, "You will come face to face with your own magnificence." Women who have given birth naturally often relate how this knowledge has helped them triumph in subsequent life challenges.

For many women, natural birth also deepens or begins a spiritual journey. Christian, Muslim, Jewish, Hindu, and pagan women, as well as women of other creeds, may find that natural birth fits with their beliefs. I have witnessed many women of faith, as well as women who belong to no religion, whose beliefs in other arenas clash significantly, come together in deep connection because of their shared understanding of the sacredness of birth. I find it virtually impossible to witness life's portals opening without contemplating all the Big Questions that spiritual traditions address: Who am I? Where did I come from? Why am I here? Sometimes, I wonder whether our high rate of anesthesia is a way of avoiding these questions.

Natural childbirth also connects our generation with the women in the hundreds of thousands of generations before us. They all (except perhaps in the last two or three generations) gave birth naturally. I was always inspired by Russian women who told me that they knew they could do it because, "My mother did it, my grandmother did it, my great-grandmother did it. Of course I can do it." If you are still thinking about whether this kind of birth is for you, ponder this: I have never met a woman who gave birth naturally and regretted it.

In the next chapters, you will prepare for the big day by visualizing your ideal birth and writing a birth plan. The first step is an exploration of why feeling safe is your number-one priority.

CHAPTER 2

FEELING SAFE

YOUR FEELINGS ABOUT SAFETY ARE THE SINGLE most important factor in how your baby's birth will unfold that are in the realm of your control.

For most of us, the mind-body connection is not something we think about often. Indeed, many of us are not comfortable with the idea that there is any real connection between the mind and the body. We live in a culture that values logic and rationality. Bodily experiences can make us uncomfortable. We have built elaborate walls between our minds and our bodies.

We may contemplate the mind-body connection occasionally during yoga class or when exercising vigorously. Perhaps chronic pain, disability, or disease inspires us to think about it. Yet nothing arouses deeper contemplation of how the mind and the body work together than pregnancy.

Pregnant women can develop a profound appreciation for their bodies. After many years of believing that we control our lives (and even our bodies), it can be a shock to watch our bodies change all on their own. We don't tell our bodies how to grow a placenta or a baby. They just know.

That your pregnant body may seem to have a life of its own does not mean there is no connection between your body and your mind. There is! Many of us intuitively understand that the emotions and thoughts of a pregnant woman influence her pregnancy and her unborn child. I can remember, for instance, the enormous outpouring of concern for me when I was eight months pregnant in New York City on September 11, 2001. Many of my friends and colleagues expressed concern that the strong emotions we were all feeling could affect a pregnant woman physically. In fact, a researcher later found that Arab-American women who were pregnant at the time of the September 11 attack gave birth to babies with significantly lower birth weights than those born to Arab-American women in the year before the attack. This was a landmark study because it was one of the first studies of discrimination and emotions that did not rely on self-reporting. Nothing could explain the difference in birth outcomes except the racial discrimination Arab Americans faced after 9/11 (Lauderdale, 2006).

Our minds and our bodies connect through our emotions. In *Ina May's Guide to Childbirth* (Gaskin, 2003), renowned midwife Ina May Gaskin gives examples that exemplify this connection: When we hear words (the mind) that embarrass us (an emotion), we blush (our body). When we watch something touching in a movie (the mind), we feel happy or sad (emotions), and we cry (our body). Emotions arise as a response to thoughts, and they manifest themselves in our bodies. The levels of our hormones increase and decrease in response to the feelings that surround every one of our thoughts and experiences. This is not just some New Age theory. It is the well-studied, scientific basis of the most common form of psychotherapy: cognitive behavioral therapy.

How does the mind-body connection affect birth? The encouraging truth is that our minds can lead the way to a satisfying, healthy birth. The flip side, though, is that fear can stop, slow, or complicate labor.

A feeling of safety, calm, and acceptance will accelerate and simplify your labor. This may sound strange or unprovable. Yet it is scientific fact. Your hormones control your labor, and your feelings control your hormones. Though many hormones are involved in the complicated dance of labor, the two most important ones to know about are adrenaline and oxytocin.

Adrenaline stops labor.
Oxytocin moves labor forward.

At the end of a pregnancy, a woman's body needs to relax and open—literally. The hormone relaxin relaxes your joints so that your pelvis can open fully. Prostaglandins relax and thin out your cervix. Your cervix, which starts out long and hard, smoothes to a thin membrane. Oxytocin courses through your blood, making you feel tender, emotional, and "ready." Finally, your body releases endorphins, morphine-like chemicals, to protect you from pain.

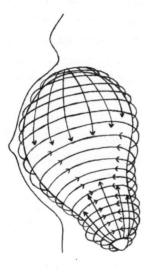

The uterine muscles contract and stretch in several different directions. During early and active labor, some muscles are squeezing inward, while others are pulling the cervix upward. When the cervix has dilated 10 centimeters, uterine muscles at the top of the uterus push downward.

Oxytocin is the hormone that contracts the uterus; it is also the hormone of feeling in love. You may be surprised to learn that labor and orgasm involve similar oxytocin-induced uterine contractions. One sensation we experience as pain, the other as pleasure. Without oxytocin, there is no labor. It's as simple as that. What shuts down oxytocin production? Fear.

When we experience fear in our mind and body, the "fight-or-flight" instinct takes over. Veterinarians know that most mammals prefer seclusion and a dark, quiet place to labor. Interruptions that cause fear may stop or slow labor. Cats that feel threatened have been known to stop labor between kittens to move to a safer place. When a mammal (and for all our rationality and language, we remain mammals!) feels threatened, adrenaline is released. Muscles tense. Oxytocin production ceases or dramatically slows. Endorphins are blocked. Organs that are nonessential to fighting or fleeing (like the uterus) receive less blood flow. This means that the baby receives less oxygen. Reduced blood flow and tense muscles increase the pain.

Doctors use oxytocin (the synthetic form has the trade name Pitocin and is often referred to as "Pit") to induce labor or to speed it up. When labor slows or stops, oxytocin is not doing its job effectively. On the one hand, it could be that the woman is not producing enough oxytocin. On the other hand, it could be that other hormones, such as adrenaline, are interfering. If adrenaline is the culprit, when the woman is given artificial oxytocin through an IV drip, she will have extraordinarily painful contractions. Her body will not produce enough pain-reducing endorphins, and it will continue to produce adrenaline in an attempt to override the oxytocin.

The writer Reinekke Lengelle interviewed obstetrician Michel Odent about the normal physiology of birth. In the 1960s and 1970s, Odent developed the maternity unit at a hospital in Pithiviers, France, where he pioneered the use of birthing pools in hospitals. Lengelle writes:

> *The needs of a woman during labor are pretty basic, and during his lecture and workshop Dr. Odent summed them up several times: privacy, safety, warmth, and darkness. These needs are pretty much what she requires to get to sleep and what will reduce the activity of the neocortex of the brain [the part of the brain that is responsible for rational, conscious thought and language]. For humans, birth is a mammalian event in which the primitive part of the brain must take center stage. When a woman feels watched, her neocortex is stimulated. When she is asked to answer questions like, "What is your address?" or "Have you had the strep B test?" her neocortex is stimulated. When the lights are bright and glaring, a cliché that lives on in hospitals everywhere, her neocortex is stimulated. If she feels threatened in any way, her labor simply slows so that, like a mammal, she can get up and find a safer place to have her baby (Lengelle, 2005).*

At Pithiviers, midwives and doctors are trained to interfere only minimally with the birth process. They keep the lights dim and the rooms warm, and they encourage women to use hydrotherapy to handle the pain of contractions. Some of these techniques can be found in the most enlightened of North American hospitals, but they are rare. Our best hospitals, the ones most serious about promoting natural birth, offer

• handheld fetal heart rate monitors to check your baby's heartbeat intermittently, so that you do not have to be hooked up to an external fetal monitor once an hour (or worse, continually!);

• birth tubs or showers for use during labor (and, if you are really lucky, for delivery, too); and

• higher-than-average rates of both vaginal and unmedicated births.

Most of us do not have the luxury of choosing an ideal hospital. One may not exist in our small town, our insurance may not allow us to choose, or a high-risk pregnancy may force us to give birth in a high-tech hospital. Often our choice of practitioner determines where we must give birth.

Yet there are ways to work within the system. Forewarned is, in fact, forearmed. Simple measures like assigning someone the task of turning out the lights each time a hospital employee leaves the room can go a long way toward improving your experience. In later chapters, we will explore what you can do to avoid triggering your own fight-or-flight response. We will look at what you have control over, externally and internally. Externally, you can make choices ahead of time about your practitioner and hospital, about your birth plan, and about hiring a doula. Internally, you can learn techniques to turn off your neocortex and find a feeling of centeredness, which will aid your labor tremendously.

The Effect of Fear on Labor: Case Studies

I have seen firsthand how fear interferes with the progress of labor. Here are three examples.

Sam

Sam arrived at her hospital birth center in active labor. Contractions were coming fast and furious; the sensations were intense. Before going into her birth room, we stopped in the clinical examination room for a quick IV dose of antibiotics. This had been planned ahead of time; Sam had tested positive for group B strep (see page 23) and had agreed to have a course of antibiotics during labor to protect her baby. Yet Sam is afraid of needles.

Her contractions had lessened in intensity as soon as we entered the birth center. When her midwife, Julie, brought out the needle, Sam's contractions completely disappeared.

After Julie had inserted the IV, we joked that perhaps we had over-reacted to Sam's contractions. She seemed to be in early labor, not active labor, after all. The next two contractions were weak. We talked about going for a walk outdoors and coming back to the birth center in a few hours.

The course of antibiotics over, we left the exam room and got about 3 feet (1 m) out the front door. Bang! We were back in business. Labor got going and didn't falter again. Looking back, we could all see the effect that needle had on Sam's labor.

Hayley

As a doula for Hayley, a twenty-three-year-old single mother, I watched in mystification as her labor stopped and started before my eyes. Because of her experiences in foster care, she was slow to trust strangers. She entered the hospital with a great deal of mistrust of people in authority. I was not surprised, therefore, that she seemed uncomfortable whenever her nurse, Sue, entered the room.

I was surprised, however, that Hayley's fears were so great that her labor virtually ceased whenever Sue (or any of the hospital staff) was nearby. The situation became almost comic. I was convinced that Hayley was in active labor by about 10 p.m. Since her contractions would significantly decrease in intensity whenever a nurse was in the room, the hospital staff believed she was in quite early labor. Hayley was declining vaginal exams because her bag of waters was broken (see page 155 for a discussion of this situation), so no one knew for sure how far along she was. Around 11 p.m. Hayley asked Sue how much longer she thought labor would last. Sue did not know that we had just struggled through several whopping contractions. As Hayley posed the question, she hardly seemed to be in labor at all.

Sue told her, "Honey, you're still in very early labor. Your baby will probably be here tomorrow or even tomorrow night. You're going to need contractions that are much closer together and much stronger than this to get the baby out!" This pattern continued for several hours. When Hayley was ready to push, the nurses were caught so off guard that they did not have time to call a doctor.

Natasha

My third example is of a young woman who gave birth in Russia, where I studied birth for a year. Generally, I was struck by the can-do attitude of most pregnant Russian women. Epidurals were not an option in the hospital where I worked. Pregnant women knew and almost universally accepted the fact that vaginal births would be accomplished without pain-relieving drugs.

Natasha, however, was an exception. She was terrified of the pain. Each contraction in her sluggish labor made her visibly more upset. Her labor had begun with her bag of waters breaking, so the hospital staff gave her twenty-four hours to give birth or at least get into active labor. Instead, she struggled through twenty-four hours of weak contractions that were irregularly spaced at eight to fifteen minutes apart. When the doctor recommended a C-section for "failure to progress," Natasha's face lit up. Her relief was palpable.

In the forty-five minutes it took to get to the surgery table, her contractions became stronger, more regular, and more frequent, until they were three to four minutes apart. She seemed to handle these stronger contractions with more self-assurance than any of those previously.

Natasha did have a C-section, but all of us who attended noticed that her labor had changed dramatically.

Using Mindfulness to Reduce Anxiety and Improve Pain Tolerance

In the last two decades, mindfulness practices have become increasingly mainstream and easy to access. According to Jon Kabat-Zinn, "Mindfulness is paying attention in a particular way: on purpose, in the present moment, and nonjudgmentally." Kabat-Zinn helped move mindfulness from the realm of religion into the scientific arena. He founded the Stress Reduction Clinic and the Center for Mindfulness in Medicine, Health Care, and Society at the University of Massachusetts. Although these meditation practices are most associated with Hinduism and Buddhism, every major religion has some connections to them, including Judaism, Christianity, and Islam.

Claims that religious leaders and their followers have made about the benefits of mindfulness practice and meditation are now being scientifically validated. For example, studies show that practitioners of mindfulness change the structure of their brain in as little as eight weeks. The "fight or flight" center, the amygdala, which is associated with fear and the body's reaction to stress, shrinks. The longer a person has practiced, the more pronounced are the effects that researchers can measure.

Here's another fascinating effect: numerous studies reveal that mindfulness helps practitioners handle pain. Though most of the studies included long-term practitioners, I was interested to discover that even a "single ten-minute mindfulness meditation intervention administered by a novice therapist can improve pain tolerance, pain threshold and decrease anxiety towards pain" (Burnett et al., 2017). There are also specific studies about the use of mindfulness to address labor pain and anxiety. Early studies are small, but promising. For example, in 2016, researchers found that a short course in mindfulness led women to feel more confident in labor, experience less depression postpartum, and use less opioid analgesia in labor (Duncan et al., 2017).

Free Mindfulness Practice Resources

Websites:

Contemplative.org This website has several useful meditations that pregnant women could try. I recommend "Breath, Sound, and Body Meditation," 12 minutes, read by Diana Winston.

Marc.ucla.edu There is a list of several audio files to choose from. Pregnant women might benefit from "Body Scan for Sleep," 13 minutes, read by Diana Winston.

Health.ucsd.edu This website offers long meditations (30 to 45 minutes) and a few short meditations (6 to 20 minutes). This is a good resource if you'd like to expand your practice and try longer sessions.

Specific Meditations:

"Mindfulness Meditation for Pain Relief" 10:37
Read by Jon Kabat-Zinn at https://goo.gl/DM3Lxn

"Connecting With Your Baby" (pregnancy meditation) 18:40
Read by Mary Maddux of Meditation Oasis at https://goo.gl/Ergvqe

This is great news for pregnant women! This easily accessible modality can help you during pregnancy and labor—and it does not have to be another drag on your "to do" list. Knowing that even small amounts of practice are beneficial is encouraging. The more you do, the better; but starting somewhere is better than nothing.

Mindfulness and hypnotherapy are not exactly the same thing; however, I find that the end goal of each practice is similar for me. Mindfulness emphasizes being very present, while hypnotherapy encourages a sort of altered mental state. Both practices induce a state in which I feel calm, relaxed, and unbothered by normal worries. Labor gets me there eventually, even if I do not use a special technique to achieve it on purpose. As a doula, I would say this is true of virtually every laboring woman I have ever attended.

If you are interested in learning more, you can check out the book *Mindful Birthing: Training the Mind, Body, and Heart for Childbirth and Beyond* by Nancy Bardacke or free online resources listed in the sidebar.

Feeling Safe: Your Number-One Priority

The feeling of safety that I am describing is that sense of peace and calm that comes over you when you know you are making the absolute right decision for yourself. This is very different from making a decision out of fear. In other words, being intuitively drawn toward a certain kind of birth experience is different from choosing a birth experience out of fear. I am sure that if you pay attention, you can distinguish between a calm feeling of self-confidence ("This is absolutely right") and an unsettling feeling of resignation ("Well, I've made the best decision possible, given all the terrible things that could go wrong").

You probably already know what makes you feel safe when you think about giving birth. You may have heard of someone's birth experience and been drawn to it instinctively. Other people's convictions can do nothing to alter such a feeling. It doesn't matter if your mother or your best friend or even your doctor feels "safer" with some line of action if you do not. Their bodies are not producing the hormones that will affect your labor.

What can you learn from Sam's, Hayley's, and Natasha's stories? I hope that you take away with you the firm belief that your feeling of safety is not only important; it is vital to a healthy labor and healthy baby. Achieving this feeling is your number-one priority as you plan for your baby's birth.

A Gentle Body Scan for Pregnancy
By Barbara Ley, Ph.D. (Duration: 10 to 15 minutes)

Consider having your partner or a friend read this out loud to you.

Please place your body in a comfortable position. You can sit upright in a chair, lie on your back, curl up on your side, or choose another position that feels comfortable and safe to you. You are also welcome to use any props that will help you relax and focus your attention on your body. Maybe you'd like to rest you head on a pillow, place a cushion behind your back or under your knees, or cover your body with a blanket. Rest your hands where they feel most natural, perhaps next to you, on your lap or belly, or above your chest.

Once you feel settled in your position, begin the body scan by bringing your attention to your breath. Begin to notice where in your body you feel your breathing the most. Perhaps you notice your chest or belly move up and down as you inhale and exhale, or perhaps you notice the air move in and out of your nostrils. Wherever you most notice your breath is fine. If, at any point, you realize that your mind has wandered away from your breath, gently—and without judging yourself for it—bring your attention back to your breath.

Now, notice how your body feels as it's breathing. Does your breathing feel fast or slow? Deep or shallow? Tight or relaxed? Can you feel the temperature of your breath as it moves in and out of your nose or mouth? Just remember that you don't have to change or control your breathing in any way. Rather, allow your body to breathe in its own way and at its own pace.

Once you feel connected to your breath, turn your attention to the surface supporting you. Notice how that surface feels against your body—perhaps you notice the back of your chair against your spine, the seat of the chair under your bottom, and your feet resting on the floor. Maybe you notice the feel of the floor or bed under your head, side, back, or legs. Also, if any part of this surface bothers your body, feel free to shift your position in a way that feels more comfortable.

Now, it's time to scan your body from head to toes. When you feel ready, slowly bring your attention to the top of your head and notice how it feels. Does it feel heavy or light? Tingly or achy? Tight or relaxed? Or maybe you don't feel anything at all. Whatever you feel on top of your head—or anywhere else in your body—is okay. Just allow the sensations to be.

Going at your own pace, move your attention down to your forehead and temples, noticing how they feel as you gently focus on them. Next, notice your eyes, nose, cheeks, jaw, and lips. You can even bring your attention to your tongue; notice where it is resting inside of your mouth and whether it feels relaxed or clenched. If your tongue—or any other part of your body for that matter—feels clenched, feel free to soften it by relaxing your muscles. Also, if focusing on a particular area of your body causes you physical or emotional distress, you can either stay with those feelings for as long as you'd like before moving on, or you can bring your attention back to your breath or another body part that feels more comfortable and safe.

Next, bring your attention to the back your head, the back of your neck, and down to your shoulders. Given that many of us carry significant stress in our shoulders and neck, you may want to spend an extra few moments noticing how they feel. Then, when you feel ready, move your awareness down the front and back of your upper arms, elbows, forearms, wrists, hands, and fingers.

Now, slowly shift your focus upward to the front of your neck and at your own pace, move your attention downward to your collarbone, chest, belly, and back. If you'd like, you can spend a few extra moments on your belly, bringing gentle awareness to your baby and to your entire abdominal area as you breathe in and out. Finally, begin to scan the lower half of your body by bringing your attention to your hips, pelvic area, buttocks, upper legs, knees, lower legs, ankles, feet, and toes.

Feel free to notice your feet and toes for as long as you'd like. You can also bring your awareness back to other areas of your body that would benefit from additional attention. For areas that feel particularly stressed or tight, you may want to try breathing into them, followed by softening them as you slowly exhale.

When you feel ready to end your body scan, slowly open your eyes, take a gentle stretch, and thank yourself for taking the time to care for your mind and body and for the mind and body of your growing baby.

Barbara L. Ley, Ph.D.
Associate Professor, Departments of Communication and Women & Gender Studies, University of Delaware, barbaraleyyoga.com

GETTING ATTACHED TO YOUR BIRTH PLAN

BIRTH PLANS—WRITTEN STATEMENTS OF HOW a mother would like her labor and delivery to occur—are controversial. Many practitioners do not like them, and for good reason. Too many birth plans are just lists of "what I do not want you to do to me." Almost every medical intervention is necessary *sometimes*, so writing a list of interventions to avoid sets women up for confrontation. Physicians have to defend the use of procedures to save a woman's or a baby's life. A birth plan written without respect for the physician's or midwife's expertise can be a source of conflict, not connection.

Another reason that birth plans are controversial is the unpredictability of birth. Birth professionals are wary that women and their partners will be disappointed if their birth experience fails to match their expectations. Well-meaning childbirth professionals tell women and their partners not to get "attached" to their birth plans. "Be flexible," they warn. "You don't know what's going to happen, you don't know how you'll react to the pain, so don't get attached to a certain way of giving birth." Many doctors and books (including one of my favorites, *Birthing from Within* [England, 1998]) go so far as discouraging women from writing down birth plans.

Yet the fact that birth is unpredictable does not mean birth plans are not useful. They are. Flexibility is important, but so is being clear about what you want.

To the call for flexibility I say, "Let the hospital be flexible! I am standing proud and firm for what I want." Wouldn't it be great if doctors were urged to be flexible to accommodate birthing women, instead of the other way around? Doctors could be trained to be flexible in delivery positions, as capable of catching a baby when the mother is on her hands and knees as when she is lying flat on her back in a bed. That's how flexibility could serve birthing women.

So here is my most important piece of advice to you: Make a birth plan, and get attached to it!

There is no other way to get what you want. In birth as in the rest of life, the clearer you are about what you want, the more likely you are to get it. Three things happen when you say out loud or write down exactly what you want:

1. You begin an internal process of aligning your actions with your goals.

2. You allow others to understand your vision and support you.

3. You become better at spotting when someone else's goals are out of alignment with yours.

Flexible is often a euphemism for *vague*. As long as you are not being specific, you and your partner or your doctor or your boss or whoever can pretend that the two of you are on the same page. The more direct and specific you are, the more direct and specific you are asking other people to be.

A good birth plan is like a good financial plan: strongly structured, yet also able to handle the unexpected. A budget is no good if it has no allowance for emergencies, and neither is a birth plan. Your birth plan should be able to accommodate the unpredictability of birth.

We may prefer not to write things down in black and white because vagueness can seem "nicer." How many of us have avoided conflict at the beauty salon only to go home and cry over a new haircut? At the hair salon and in the hospital, none of us enjoys confrontation. The price that we may pay for being nice, however, is missing out on the birth experience that we truly want. In interviews and on Internet sites, hundreds of women tell about going along with something with which they disagreed during labor because they felt uncomfortable coming into conflict with their medical provider or with their partner. Some of the stories are heart-wrenching, since the women so clearly regret their decisions.

Being clear about what we want can sometimes lead to confrontation. But it can often lead to getting what we want.

Getting Attached

Here's the risk: getting attached to your birth plan means that you will feel disappointed if you don't get what you've decided you want. But feeling disappointment can be healthy and life-enhancing. Not getting what we want in life *is* disappointing. Isn't it always better to strive and fall short than to never strive at all? Since when has it become unacceptable to feel sadness, disappointment, or anger? Repressing strong emotions like disappointment is a normal reflex in North America and some parts of western Europe. Not coincidentally, these are the same places where women most often repress pain in childbirth.

Getting attached to your birth plan, like getting attached to anything or anyone in your life, makes you vulnerable. You are, indeed, risking not getting what you want. The alternative is virtually ensuring that you don't get what you want by leaving events to chance.

When I ended up with an epidural and a C-section, I was extremely disappointed. Even though I knew in my heart that the intervention had saved my baby's life, I was still angry and sad. Acknowledging and appropriately expressing these feelings seems infinitely more appealing to me than trying to be flexible and not caring too deeply how I gave birth.

North Americans are often confused by feeling more than one emotion at the same time. When our obstetricians say, "You don't want to be disappointed," they may assume that it is impossible to hold disappointment in our hearts together with joy at the birth of a healthy newborn. My experience as a birthing woman and a doula says otherwise. The paradox of being happy and sad about birth seems more natural and appropriate to me than a steady state of one emotion.

Women who are upset about their birth experiences but who did not write birth plans often say, "If only I had known" or, "If only I had prepared." In contrast, mothers who prepare for a natural birth and write birth plans but end up with necessary interventions do not have to blame themselves for lack of preparation. They are free to mourn without self-recrimination.

Three Steps to an Effective Birth Plan

I recommend a triple-layer process for writing a birth plan: Dream It, Plan It, Write It.

Step 1: Dream the birth.

Step 2: Plan the whole birth, not just the medical parts.

Step 3: Write the medical birth plan to share with your team.

At the end, you should have two documents: one that describes your whole birth plan, and one that describes mostly the medical parts of your birth plan. The whole birth plan is for you, your partner, and anyone else whom you may want to include. This plan is usually long and detailed. The medical birth plan is far shorter and more concise. You can hand it to an obstetrician or a labor-and-delivery nurse, and that person will understand your preferences in just a few seconds.

Most of the birth-plan forms offered on websites are checklists of interventions that you may want to avoid. These forms are sometimes useful, yet a birth plan that grows out of a positive vision of a wonderful birth is much more attractive and less likely to raise the hackles of hospital personnel.

Step 1 involves exercises to discover your ideal birth. As you will read, an ideal birth is not limited by reality. You can dream about your grandmother being in the room even if she passed away some years ago. It's all right if your ideal birth would take place in the ocean—even if you live in Nebraska. It's the process of acknowledging your deepest desires that will help you.

You add reality to the mix in step 2. After visualizing a perfect birth, you ask yourself which elements of that dream are important to include in the real birth. Many of these elements will have nothing to do with your obstetrical care, so you won't need to include them on the short form that you give to your team. Through this process, however, many women realize that the absence of medical intervention underlies their entire birth vision. When they finally sit down for step 3, writing a birth plan to share with their team, they can focus on the areas that are most important.

Step 1: Dream It

The first step in writing a birth plan is to dream.

Let go of all the "shoulds" and pressing realities that circumscribe your choices. Let yourself visualize the perfect, ideal birth for you. Trust that later you can add in reality. Right now, let loose your feelings and your imagination. It's OK to invoke magic in your dream birth. Think through all the stages of labor: early, active, pushing the baby into the world, and the first hour with your new baby (if your understanding of these stages is hazy, see Chapter Six). Get specific about the details.

It's important to allow yourself to dream without anxiety. Put all concerns about safety aside. In your ideal birth, you are in perfect health, and you have just the amount of stamina that you need.

Though you have decided to give birth in a hospital, I recommend that you watch videos of out-of-hospital births to stimulate your most authentic birth vision. We have seen birth only one way: a woman lies in a brightly lit hospital room, panting and squeezing her partner's hand while a doctor sits between her legs at the foot of a bed. We have seen this Hollywood version of birth too many times to conjure any other image on our own. It is how 99 percent of women on the cable television show *A Baby Story* give birth. It is probably how your mother and your grandmother gave birth. It is probably how most of your friends have given birth.

It is not how most women in the world give birth.

Though you will give birth in a hospital, your dream birth may not be in a hospital or even indoors at all. Turn off the mainstream media to find your own true, authentic image. Your dream birth will inspire your real birth experience.

Ask your life partner, if you have one, to do this exercise, too. Your partner's dreams and visions may influence what you ultimately decide to do. Even if your visions clash, sharing them will be the first step toward integration. This process can be powerfully connecting. If you have any concerns that your partner's vision will overpower your own, I recommend that you complete these exercises alone or with another trusted person before you talk to your life partner. Getting to the heart of what you need and want is most important at this stage.

Here are two examples of "dream births" to get your creative juices flowing. Ruth Ann's and Zafira's dream births are examples of using fantasy to reach one's truest, deepest desires. It might be impossible for them to realize their dreams exactly as described, yet their fantasies tell these two very different women what is really important to them.

Ruth Ann's Dream Birth

Ruth Ann's Labor Ruth Ann fantasizes about laboring on a stretch of ocean beach near Moss Beach, California, that is devoid of houses and development, where seals often rest on rocks, and whales and dolphins also visit. She imagines starting labor in the late afternoon, packing a picnic with her husband, and walking from their apartment to the beach. She envisions pacing on the sand barefoot as the contractions get stronger, watching the sun setting, hearing the birds and the ocean waves, and concentrating during contractions on her footprints in the sand.

Ruth Ann's Delivery When the contractions build to the point of imminent birth, Ruth Ann's perfect location changes. She imagines a break in the pain. She and her husband are magically transported to a lake at the top of a mountain. At the mountaintop her sisters, girl-friends, and a beloved aunt (who is actually deceased) are waiting for her. The pain of labor subsides long enough for her to greet them all. Then, by moon- and starlight, they all enter the lake. Ruth Ann's husband and women friends support her body. The baby is born in the water into a circle of loving arms.

Ruth Ann's First Hour with Her Baby The location changes again. Magically, Ruth Ann and her husband are instantly transported back to their home. They spend the first hours postpartum cocooned in bed with the new baby. All their helpers (midwife, sisters, aunt, friends) are busy cooking in the kitchen. Smells of Italian food waft up the stairs.

If you are having trouble imagining yourself in other places or other positions, check out these videos for inspiration:

Birth into Being: The Russian Waterbirth Experience, produced by Barbara Harper in 1999 and available at www.birthintobeing.com (Wilsonville, OR: Global Maternal Child Health Association; 28 minutes). With stirring sequences of birth in the sea, this inspiring video will stretch your imagination about what is possible.

Birth in the Squatting Position, available from www.birthworks.org or www.1cascade.com and also on YouTube. This beautiful, inspiring ten-minute video from Brazil leaves indelible images of strong, capable, upright birthing women.

Zafira's Dream Birth

Zafira's Labor Zafira imagines laboring by herself at home. She does not want her husband nearby. He would be too distracting. When labor becomes intense, she wants her mother and sister to arrive in her mother's car and drive her to the hospital. She imagines gaining confidence from her mother's love and example (she has birthed many children "without complaining," says Zafira) and the presence of her sister, who gave birth the year before. Zafira imagines arriving at the hospital to a room that is dark and cool and bypassing the usual medical tests.

Zafira's Delivery Zafira imagines giving birth in the dark, cozy hospital room. The doctors and nurses do not talk to her much or interfere with the natural process of labor. She cannot see their faces clearly because they are present only to give a sense of safety, not to interact with her. She imagines squatting at the edge of the bed, using the squat bar, to give birth. As soon as the baby is born, her husband is allowed into the room. The baby hears the father's voice before any other, reciting a meaningful line from the Koran and calling the baby by name.

Zafira's First Hour with Her Baby Zafira's baby is held and touched only by loving relatives, not by hospital staff. Zafira's mother and sister stay close by, to give her drinks and help dress the baby in special clothes. Zafira's mother, instead of a nurse, washes the baby after the birth. Her mother and sister offer help with breastfeeding. Her husband does something wonderful and surprising to commemorate the day that their first child was born.

Now, it's your turn. You can read the questions in the next section and answer them in your mind, or you can write down your answers. There's no right or wrong way to do this exercise.

Step 2: Plan It

Now that you've dreamed into the future, you can start to make a birth plan. In this step, you will identify what is most meaningful in your dream birth so that you can include those elements in your plan. After reflecting on your ideal birth, you will examine some events from your past. Finally, you will write a whole birth plan.

Reflect on Your Ideal Birth

Many extroverts need to talk out loud before writing their plan; introverts may be able to reflect inwardly. Either in discussion or in contemplation, you can identify the elements of a safe, wonderful, joyous birth event.

When Ruth Ann talked with her best friend about her upcoming labor, they realized that being connected to nature, and in particular to water, was very important to her. Ruth Ann could imagine feeling centered and peaceful during labor if she could hear running water and immerse herself in a bathtub. Ruth Ann originally planned to use the hospital closest to her home, but after thinking things through, she decided to switch to a hospital about half an hour away because the second hospital had whirlpool tubs. Ruth Ann also decided to pack a recording of nature sounds to play during labor. When her best friend showed up at the birth, she brought with her a small, plug-in waterfall.

Your Dream Birth

Some questions to get you started

1. If you could labor and deliver your baby anywhere in the world and in any setting, without having to worry about safety, where would your fantasy birth take place? Would you like to be in one place for the whole experience? Or would different parts of the experience feel right in different settings?

2. Describe each stage of labor in your dream birth.
   a. Early labor:
      Where are you?
      Who is with you?
      What do you hear?
      What do you see?
      What do you smell?
      What do you feel?
      What or who helps you in this place to feel calm?

   b. Active labor:
      Where are you?
      Who is with you?
      What do you hear?
      What do you see?
      What do you smell?
      What do you feel?
      What or who helps you in this place to feel calm?

   c. Pushing:
      Where are you?
      Who is with you?
      What do you hear?

What do you see?

What do you smell?

What do you feel?

What or who helps you in this place to feel calm?

d. First hour of the baby's life:

Where are you?

Who is with you?

What do you hear?

What do you see?

What do you smell?

What do you feel?

What or who helps you in this place to feel calm?

3. When you are in pain, what types of personal comforts (a quiet room, heat, cold, words spoken, and so on) do you like to use?

4. Where do you hold tension in your body, and what helps you let it go?

5. What is your biggest fear about labor and delivery? What helps relieve this fear? (If this question feels overwhelming, please think about getting extra help in this process. Doulas are often a good, safe place to start. If you would benefit from specific therapies to reduce fear, doulas can usually recommend local practitioners such as psychotherapists or hypnotists. Some women have reported good results with a psychotherapeutic treatment called EMDR, or Eye Movement Desensitization and Reprocessing. Women who have heard horrific birth stories or who have traumatic histories may need help to process their fears.)

Identify the Meaningful Elements of Your Dream

As you reflect on your ideal birth, ask yourself what elements you can incorporate into your real birth plan. What are the sights, sounds, and smells that you would like to experience? If there are unrealistic parts of your ideal birth, are there ways to incorporate meaningful symbols?

For instance, Ruth Ann knew that she could not invite her deceased aunt to her birth, but she wanted to invoke her love and presence. So she wrote a long letter to her cousin, her aunt's daughter, detailing her wish that her aunt could be there and explaining how much her aunt had meant to her. In response, her cousin sent her the clothes that her mother had first worn as a baby. These were the clothes in which Ruth Ann dressed her baby soon after birth.

For Extroverts

Talk to a friend when you're ready to reflect on your ideal birth. Pick a person with whom you feel safe discussing your deepest fears and desires, someone who can listen without judgment. Often, the people who are closest to us (our life partners, mothers, sisters, and even best friends) have trouble doing this. In this case, I recommend that you pick a more neutral person in your life for this exercise. When it is done, you can talk to your loved ones with more self-awareness.

In reviewing her dream birth, Zafira realized how important it was to her to incorporate her religious traditions into her birth plan. So she asked her mother to bring the well-worn family copy of the Koran to the hospital. I've been at births that included heirloom quilts and pictures of a blooming rose. Many families plan to bake a birthday cake for the baby when the mother begins early labor or to ask relatives to do so while they are at the hospital.

What will make your baby's birth more meaningful and special to you?

Whom to Invite

For many women, the questions of whom to invite and how much to involve them are sticking points. I ask you to get in touch with your wisest inner self to answer these questions. Ask yourself if you will feel more joyful and supported if a certain person is with you at the birth. If you know, deep inside, that you will feel inhibited, criticized, or upset in any way because of this person's presence, acknowledge that this is true. If this person will have a close relationship with your baby, you can plan to involve the person in your baby's life in a way that also honors *you*. Perhaps this is the right person to host the baby's name ceremony or christening party. There are many creative ways to include friends or relatives in your child's life without inviting them to the birth.

Ruth Ann decided to share her dream birth with her sisters and closest girlfriends. When Ruth Ann reflected on her wedding day, she remembered that she had always pictured getting her hair and nails done together with her three sisters and three of her friends from high school. She had hoped they would all get into their dresses together and giggle their way through the morning. Somehow, she neglected to tell them of her hopes, and so she ended up getting ready the morning of her wedding without them.

She did not want to repeat this mistake at the birth. This time, she decided to be clear and direct about what she envisioned. She invited her sisters and friends to come to the hospital and be "on call" in the waiting room in case she needed their presence and support during labor, but she wanted them to know ahead of time that she was not necessarily inviting them to participate in the whole process. Ruth Ann remembers:

> When I went on the hospital tour, there was a woman in labor who was walking around the hospital hallways, and every time she went around the hallway, she would stop in the waiting room and chat with her family. There were at least ten people in there! Then she'd get a contraction and keep on walking down the hallway with her husband. Her family went back to watching TV. That looked great to me. I would love knowing that my sisters and friends were close by, that I could talk to them whenever I wanted to just by going down the hallway. But I also know I want to be with just Jason and the new baby when it is first born.

One of her sisters was not happy about this arrangement. She was insulted that Ruth Ann was inviting so many other people to the birth and even threatened not to come. Ruth Ann considered "uninviting" her, but she really wanted her there. In the end, her sister did show up at the hospital, and Ruth Ann felt touched and happy that her sister overcame her initial reluctance to support her plan.

Though Ruth Ann risked conflict with her sister, her careful analysis of her ideal birth and past experiences allowed her to create the birth experience she wanted.

Lessons from Your Past

Now is your opportunity to contemplate past rites of passage in your life. This sort of reflection often helps us realize what obstacles we face within ourselves or within our relationships. There's no sense in repeating the problems you've faced before. In step 2, you are planning your baby's whole birth, not just the medical parts.

I will offer several areas of reflection. You can choose to focus on as many or as few of these areas as you'd like. In the end, by combining the insights you've gained from the previous step with reflections on your past, you will be able to plan a birth and create a document that reflects your core birth values.

A Previous Birth

If you have already had a baby, you will naturally be thinking a lot about your past birth experience as you prepare to give birth this time. If you had a wonderful experience the first time, you probably have confidence that you can do it again. If the previous birth was not so wonderful, you need to resolve any feelings from the past so you can free yourself to be in the moment, fully present at the new birth.

Some women who have had inspiring first births find themselves worried that their luck will run out. The coming birth might seem doomed. If this is how you feel, you can benefit from the advice in this section, too.

One of the beautiful aspects of being human is that we can learn from the past and plan the future. But, as Richard Layard reports in

Happiness: Lessons from a New Science (2005), we are not always talented at learning the right lessons from our past. We get stuck believing that whatever happened last is what is going to happen next. That's why people sell stocks when the prices are going down and buy when they are going up.

If you live in North America, your previous labor probably included some or many medical interventions. These days, one out of every three women experiences the ultimate medical intervention: a cesarean section. If you are reading this book, you have probably decided that this medicalized birth experience is not what you want to repeat. You may have gone to the hospital the first time without knowing much about what to expect. Or you may have planned a natural birth, but it didn't happen. Either way, you have a lot of emotions about your first labor.

You are probably worried that negative experiences from the past will repeat themselves. How do you learn from the past and move on?

1. By delving deeply into your feelings about the past birth experience

2. By acknowledging the uniqueness of this child and this birth

3. By seeking out women's stories about how different one birth can be from the next

Acknowledge your feelings. Your feelings about the past birth are real. You can't talk yourself out of them. You know this, because you've probably tried.

I've worked with women whose fears from previous births function in two different ways. The first is a straightforward fear of reexperiencing something difficult or traumatic. The second is more complicated. Women can fear the feelings of guilt or disappointment that they remember from a previous birth. Fear of feeling guilty can prevent women from planning a natural birth again. They don't want to reexperience the disappointment of not achieving their goals.

If you experienced something difficult in a previous birth, you are understandably worried about it happening again. Perhaps your labor plateaued when your cervix had dilated to 6 centimeters, and you ended up with Pitocin and an epidural. You will naturally worry during your pregnancy and during your labor that the same thing will occur again. Can you imagine the rush of fear you will feel when your caregiver does a vaginal exam in labor and tells you that you are at 6 centimeters? Or perhaps the first time around you made it to "transition" (see pages 117 to 118) and you cried out in great fear, "I can't do this anymore! Help me!" and your partner called the nurse to order an epidural. In this case, you are worried that this time you will run out of internal reserves to make it through those last 2 centimeters on your own.

If you acknowledge that these fears are real, you can plan for difficult moments. You can tell your support team exactly what you want to hear at these times. You can plan to play a particular recorded song that will inspire you. You can plan to let yourself cry. In other words, it is normal and natural to worry that you will repeat your previous experience, but this doesn't mean you can't accept your fear and move on. It's a powerful paradox: on the one hand, you can feel fear about repeating the past, and on the other hand, you can feel hope about doing things differently this time.

It is relatively common in our country to experience emotional trauma in labor. Many women undergo painful interventions in the birth process because their care providers are worried about the baby. In labor, with strong hormones flowing through her blood, a mother hears a doctor say, "I'm worried about your baby's low heart rate," and she experiences the shock of any mother whose child teeters on the edge of death. In the grip of such terror, women will agree to medical interventions to "save" the baby. Later, such a mother may come to understand that her baby was not as close to danger as she thought, but her emotional memory and her bodily memory don't always match her intellectual understanding of the situation. Pregnant again, such a woman may feel panic-stricken about labor. If this is the case for you, please read Chapter Five, "Extra Support for Special Circumstances." You are likely to need extra support and extra care during labor. The good news is that research shows that having a natural birth after such a trauma can be wonderfully healing (Sperlich & Seng, 2008).

Finally, some of us get hobbled by our fear of being disappointed again. A woman I know named Jill planned a natural birth the first time around but ended up with an epidural after thirty-six hours of active labor. When she got the epidural, she felt intense relief. She could finally rest, after seemingly endless pain. After the birth, she felt guilty not only that she had accepted an epidural, but also that she had felt relief and happiness. She felt guilty that she was not "committed enough" to natural birth. She told herself that if she had been committed, she would have felt disappointed, not relieved, when she received the epidural.

When she got pregnant a second time, she went out of her way to avoid planning a natural birth. She was determined to be open to whatever might happen, especially another long labor that might leave her exhausted. Since avoiding medications in American hospitals requires strong determination, it is not surprising that she ended up with an epidural in her second labor. Her second labor was significantly shorter than her first, and she got the epidural this time when she was in transition. Her baby was born about forty minutes later.

She had avoided planning a natural birth the second time around to forestall feelings of guilt. Ironically, she experienced feelings of guilt, sadness, and disappointment anyway. Days after the birth, she cried about her decision to accept an epidural. "I was so close," she said, "but I was scared of having hours to go." She had been so careful to be open to an epidural that her midwife and her partner felt comfortable offering it to her. Avoiding guilt became more important than achieving her heart's desire. In the end, she did not avoid the guilt. And she still didn't get the birth she wanted.

Focus on *this* birth. Most of us blame our own bodies for "failure" in labor. We forget that labor is a social dance with a lot of dancers. There is the mother, of course, and there is the baby. Each baby is different. Just a slight tilt of the baby's head to one side can make all the difference between a thirty-six-hour labor and a ten-hour labor. Our support team and caregivers and nurses are all part of the dance. Sometimes their well-meaning comments can drain us of resolve and confidence. We must do our best to make sure our team is on board with our plan.

Seek out stories. While we fixate on a previous birth, we can easily discount the stories of the women around us who say, "My last labor was *so* different from the one before!" Instead of holding on to the idea that events will repeat themselves, we can tune our antennae to the birth stories that give us a different message. As statistics and anecdotes tell us, complications in a first labor are highly unlikely to recur. Especially inspiring are stories from women who had unsatisfying first labors but went on to have wonderful second labors. Ask such women what they did differently the second time. What changed?

Past Rituals

Before you finalize your birth plan according to your ideal birth and, possibly, your reflections on a past birth, I encourage you to reflect on a past ritual from your life. As the anthropologist Robbie Davis-Floyd points out, giving birth is more than a physical experience; it is also an event that marks a significant life transition. She wrote an entire book on this topic, *Birth as an American Rite of Passage* (2004). From this perspective, birth belongs in the same category as life events such as baptisms, bar and bat mitzvahs, weddings, graduations, retirements, and funerals. These moments divide our lives into "before" and "after." As we move from one stage of life into the next, we are transformed.

Women whom I interviewed for this book often spontaneously told me stories about important ritual occasions in their lives. They described their weddings, or the funeral of a grandparent, or Christmas dinner with in-laws, or attending a niece's kindergarten graduation. Their stories made it clear that threads of each family's tapestry somehow were woven into pregnancies and births, for better or worse. Family conflicts about power, money, time, and energy often erupt around ritual occasions. At the same time, these events connect people in deep, meaningful ways.

There are many rituals involved in hospital birth over which you will have little control. Yet there are many over which you do have control. You can plan to incorporate rituals into your labor and birth that will enhance your experience. Such details can make a big difference.

I am not suggesting, however, that rituals such as lighting candles can replace the hard work of labor. My friend Amy, in Southern California, is skeptical of women who put great effort into planning aromatherapy for birth but who do not spend time preparing for the physical marathon of labor. She is right. Labor, even if it is scented with peppermint, is demanding. The point is to learn about yourself and apply what you can.

One of the most powerful lessons we can learn from past rituals is how well we have created what we want. When you look back at a ritual event that you orchestrated, are you filled with delight and wonder at your creation? If so, you have probably developed the talent of asking yourself what you want and manifesting your heart's desire. You probably know how to talk to your friends and relatives about what you want in a way that is inclusive and not alienating, but that also ensures you will feel good about what you create. You do not let other people's ideas about what "should" happen run your show.

Most of us are still learning how to do this. Our memories of past ceremonies and holidays can be bittersweet. Women often feel trapped in a people-pleasing role. We may find it difficult to stand up for what we truly want, even at the most precious moments of our lives. You can easily tell when this has happened to you because the memory of an event brings up resentment. This useful feeling points the way toward what you want, but you have to take the time to listen to it.

If you were left feeling resentful after a ritual event, what can you learn about yourself and what you need for your birth plan? Were there areas of your holiday or your ceremony to which you gave less thought or attention than you later wished you had? If so, what can you do during your pregnancy that will help you feel better prepared for the birth?

Ask yourself whether anything likely to happen during your labor might make you feel resentful or fill you with regret afterward. Can you keep this thing from happening? If so, change your birth plan to reflect what you really want.

Here are some examples of connections women have found between past rites of passage and their upcoming labors:

Ruth Ann recalled the special memory from her wedding of driving from the church to the reception hall with her new husband. They were alone together for about fifteen minutes, and they didn't say many words to each other. But they kept looking at each other and smiling.

As Ruth Ann planned her baby's birth, she wanted to make sure that she and Jason would have those "special fifteen minutes" to bond with their new baby. She talked to her obstetrician with great conviction about having this bonding time immediately after the birth. Though her doctor said the request was unusual, she agreed to it. (You can see Ruth Ann's full birth plan on pages 50 and 51.)

When Laura was planning her wedding, it was very important to her that the ceremony be outdoors, in nature. She ended up being married near a lake. Not surprisingly, her dream birth was also outdoors and near a lake. She felt sure that she wanted to be connected to nature during her labor and that using water during labor would help her. She spent early labor outdoors in sunshine. She used a shower and a bath for about two hours of her labor, and she says they were the "best two hours of the whole thing. I was able to doze off between contractions, and the pain was much more manageable when I was in water."

On the day Lily was to graduate from medical school, she was given a piece of advice by a friend. The day would go by in a blur, the friend said, so Lily should pick one moment to look around and consciously fix the moment in her memory. Lily asked her husband to help her do the same thing in birth. She was grateful that she was able to take a clear, happy memory snapshot of an otherwise blurry-feeling labor.

Susan confided that she still carried a grudge about how overbearing her mother had been during the planning for her wedding. At first, Susan planned to invite her mother to her labor. Upon reflection about her wedding, though, she became aware that "doing the right thing" by inviting her mother would probably have a negative effect on her labor. She knew that her mother might try to come even if uninvited, so she appointed a friend as gatekeeper. In fact, her mother did try to crash the birth, and her friend had to ask her firmly to leave.

Zafira, whose birth plan is described on page 52, believes that marriage and birth are sacred events. For her, the religious meanings of these events are much more important than the medical or legal meanings. Her wedding ceremony was designed with traditional religious rituals. At her baby's birth, she asked the medical staff to ensure that the first words her baby would hear upon entering the world would be words of praise for God.

Some questions to get you started

Pick one ritual event (Thanksgiving or your wedding, for example), and answer the following questions about it. You can do this several times, with different events.

1. What do you remember most vividly from the event?

2. What moment do you treasure most in your memory?

3. What do you most regret?

4. Whose presence made the event extra-special?

5. Whose presence made the event extra-stressful?

6. When you give others advice about how to plan such an event, what do you tell them?

7. How did you handle decision making when something did not go as planned (for instance, your flowers arrived late or rain threatened an outdoor ceremony)?

8. If you could do it all over again, what would you change and what would you keep the same?

Tests of Your Endurance and Strength

Take time to reflect on how you have handled mental, physical, and emotional endurance tests in your life up to this point. Just like social rituals, such trials give us a wealth of information about our strengths and weaknesses.

Women who have tested themselves through feats of physical endurance—such as marathons, half marathons, triathlons, and long-distance cycling events—or who play sports regularly can look to these experiences for strength and inspiration.

But what if you are a dyed-in-the-wool couch potato who avoids the gym and any strenuous exercise whatsoever? You, too, have probably experienced feats of endurance. For instance, did you ever write a long paper or a thesis? Did you attend college while holding down two jobs? Have you ever busted your patootie on a project at work? Have you put together a car out of scrap parts? Have you written and rewritten a song for guitar a million times until it was perfect? These are all accomplishments that require significant concentration, dedication, and an ability to get "in the flow."

Sujutha's Story: Spinning Through Labor

When I started Spinning, a kind of group exercise on stationary bicycles, I had no idea how well it would prepare me for giving birth. According to my instructor, sprints were useful ways to improve our speed and to push our hearts, lungs, and muscles a bit further. He told us to give each sprint everything we had. He warned us that we would start to feel fatigued about fifteen seconds into the sprint, and that after about forty-five seconds, our bodies would naturally start to slow down. We were supposed to try to fight this natural slow-down. We completed each sprint with nothing left to give. Later, I recognized this pattern in labor. It was exactly how a contraction felt!

I felt silly the first time I did sprints in Spinning class, while listening to my friends shout, "Go, Suji, go! You can do it!" and, "You're kicking butt! Push it, push it, push it!" But I must say that I was soon addicted to the encouragement. There was nothing like feeling exhausted, ready to give up, and hearing the person next to me say, "Don't stop now! You can do it! Just ten more seconds! Come on! Go harder, give it all you've got!" It gave me that extra oomph. I amazed myself by consistently finding strength I didn't know I had to push just a little bit harder at the end.

I also learned to moan and groan in company. Prior to doing Spinning sprints, I had gone to many yoga and aerobics classes. I sweated my way through them all silently.

"Roar!" commanded our Spinning instructor. At first, I remained silent, just listening to everyone else. But, of course, I was quickly found out. I felt ridiculous. The only noises I could think to make while Spinning sounded embarrassingly like the noises I make in bed. How could I share those in polite company? But, as I was on the spot, I was too embarrassed not to join in. Everyone else had been happily making fools of themselves, and it was impolite not to participate. So I did. And it was great! Making noises helped me gain access to that extra bit of strength, deep down in my gut.

Sprints and labor contractions have a lot in common. I am eternally grateful for Trainer Jack's lesson: I can give a sprint—or a contraction—my all and be completely spent at the end of sixty seconds. Then, if I rest for sixty seconds, I can find the strength to do it again! And again. And again.

Flow is different from effort. Some athletes assume that their physical fitness will enable them to endure childbirth pain. They think they can muscle their way through labor. Strength and endurance are invaluable tools, but the advantage of flow is that it marries strength with relaxation.

In Sujatha's story, she compares her first natural birth experience to cycling. She found that practicing physical sprints helped her in labor. She was used to being physically drained at the end of a sixty-second sprint, but she knew that she could trust her body to recoup its strength to repeat the sprint just a minute later. Effort and relaxation are equally important. If you can remember how you accomplished your mental or physical feats of endurance, you can access those remarkable parts of yourself for birth.

Some questions to get you started

1. What physical activity have you done that took the most out of you? That you are most proud of? That required the most endurance?

2. What mental activity have you done that took the most out of you? That you are most proud of? That required the most endurance?

3. List five ways that you can find that extra oomph, that little bit of stamina left in you when you thought you had nothing left to give.

4. Where do your thoughts go when you are doing something physical that you want to do but that is painful in some way? What do you think about? What do you say to yourself?

5. Does the thought of physical trial and accomplishment thrill you or scare you or both?

6. What helps you relax the most? Describe the most relaxing experience of your life.

7. Describe three activities you do that "take you out of yourself" and make the passing of time seem instantaneous.

Step 3: Write It

The Whole Birth Plan

After you've analyzed your dream birth and reflected on any previous birth experience, a social ritual, and a feat of endurance from your past, you're ready to write your "whole birth" birth plan. This is different from the birth plan you will share with your medical caregivers, which you will write next. Your plan can be as long or as short as you'd like. You will have enough insight now to answer these important questions:

1. What elements in your environment are most conducive to allowing you to freely express yourself without inhibition?

2. What elements in your environment help you achieve a feeling of peace?

3. What elements in your environment allow you to feel most in control?

4. What elements in your environment allow you to look deeply inward, for depths you have never reached before?

5. Who should be at your baby's birth?

6. Who has important relationships with you and the new baby? How will you best honor these relationships and also honor your needs during labor?

7. How can you set up the birth room to provide the sights, sounds, and smells that you want to experience?

The Birth Plan for the Hospital

You are now ready to write the birth plan that you will share with your medical caregiver and birth team. This document will arise out of your positive vision of the birth. To be effective, the plan should be succinct and easy to read, even in just a few minutes (which may be all your nurse can spare when you arrive at the hospital ready to push). Because you are attempting to avoid many of the interventions that nurses and doctors consider routine, make sure that your plan sounds polite, respectful, and positive.

I offer for your consideration the possibility of a two-sentence birth plan: "Dear Birth Team: Please help me achieve the most natural birth possible. I'm so grateful for everyone who is helping us on this wonderful day. Sincerely, [your name]."

This simple birth plan has a number of advantages. First, it respects the expertise of the birth team. Your doctor or midwife spent thousands of hours learning about birth. Do you think she wants you to decide which interventions are acceptable and which are not? To your caregiver, an episiotomy is a medical decision, not a personal preference.

Many websites offer checklist birth plans. Usually, you check off the interventions that you want to avoid. Unfortunately, many nurses and doctors react negatively to such plans. Many go so far as to say, "As soon as I see one of those, I know we're headed for a C-section."

The two-sentence birth plan, in contrast, invites your team to be on board with your birthing philosophy, not with specific decisions. Virtually every nurse and doctor understand from the first sentence that you are hoping to avoid pain medications, Pitocin, and a C-section, and that you are willing to work hard. The two-sentence plan orients the team toward the overall experience you are hoping to have and away from arguments about specific procedures.

Still, the two-sentence plan may be too concise. To expand, I encourage you to focus on the areas that matter the most to you. For most women, I recommend including a sentence or two about each of the following areas, which have the most potential to affect your experience:

1. Beginning labor naturally, even if you pass your due date and even if your bag of waters breaks before contractions begin
2. Delaying the offer of pain medication until you ask for it
3. Holding your baby immediately after birth

Wherever possible, I recommend that you use positive rather than negative statements. For example, "I would like to begin labor naturally" is better than "I do not want Pitocin."

In addition, you should add anything that is unique to your situation. For instance, Ruth Ann's plan emphasized her desire to use hydrotherapy during labor, and Zafira's plan included her desire to respect the baby and the birthing space as holy. The plans that Ruth Ann and Zafira distributed to their teams appear on pages 66–68.

Visual Birth Plans

In the last few years, a new kind of birth plan has emerged and become very popular: a visual birth plan. The idea is that a visual birth plan is easy for hospital staff to understand quickly without having to read a lot of text. Such a plan is best for a caregiver or hospital that you fear will not take the time to really read and pay attention to a more traditional birth plan. The visual nature and speed of such a plan is ideal for such caregivers or hospitals.

I think the idea of a visual representation of your desires is a wonderful impulse; however, I am not convinced that most apps go beyond the "checklist" formula of other online birth plans. They give an illusion of being "customized" (you chose the images/buttons that are included, after all), but in reality, the hard work of distilling what is important *to you* may not be included in such a plan.

In the end, I am not sure whether a pastel square with an icon of a woman and a pair of scissors and the words *no episiotomy* really carries the same weight as a thoughtful sentence on a birth plan such as this one: "I hope to use warm compresses and position changes to avoid tearing; if I will tear, I'd prefer to tear naturally." One feels like fast food to me and the other feels like a home-cooked meal.

If you like the idea of a visual birth plan, I encourage you to consider making your own. Of course, not everyone will feel confident about drawing or visually representing themselves that way. But, if you do enjoy drawing or making art other ways, this is an excellent opportunity to make a very meaningful, useful, and beautiful document.

If you decide to use an app or online program, you can still *customize* your printout with your own words handwritten on the page. Highlight what is most important to you in some way. Otherwise, the list of icons can flatten out your preferences and make them all look equally important. I hope that the triple-layer birth plan process leads you to an attractive, easy-to-understand final document, written, visual, or a combination, that you will feel proud to hand to your caregivers.

Planning for an Unexpected Cesarean

This book is designed to help you avoid an unnecessary cesarean. There are far too many cesareans performed worldwide every year. In the United States, roughly one in three births ends in surgery; in some places in the world, percentages in big cities reach into the 70 or 80 percent range. Hopefully, the tools and skills you will build will allow you to avoid an unnecessary C-section.

That said, I am not superstitious about planning for an unexpected cesarean. It's smart to plan now, when you have time to research and ask questions. In the event that your baby needs a cesarean for real, valid medical reasons, it will be too late to get online and read about cesareans. Don't let your fear of an undesired outcome keep you from being informed.

The truth is that sometimes our babies, and, indeed, sometimes our own bodies, need cesareans. In a perfect medical environment, we think that about 10 percent (perhaps 8 percent, perhaps 15 percent) of births would be performed by cesarean section. Though the idea of such a birth experience may be frightening, I know from years of attending births that most women who plan well for a natural, vaginal birth do not end up frightened if their babies need a surgical birth. Because of their planning, they know, deep in their hearts, that they needed the surgery. When a woman is plagued with doubts about a possibly unnecessary cesarean, it can feel genuinely awful—indeed, traumatic—for a long time. But women who are certain of the choices that they made, who felt supported all the way through pregnancy and labor and surgery, do not have to second-guess themselves for the rest of their lives.

I invite you to research "gentle cesareans," also called "family-centered cesareans," online and to ask questions of your caregiver about what would be possible in this scenario. Then, if you'd like, you can include a few of these bullet points on your birth plan. However, it's more important that you do your research, know what you want, and have conversations during pregnancy with your caregiver than that every single preference gets put down on your birth plan.

A few things to consider include the following:

• **Support People**

Can you bring more than one support person with you into the operating room? Bringing a doula into the OR can often help you *and your partner* feel calm during a potentially scary time. Doulas across the United States and Canada report that more and more hospitals understand the benefits of their presence at cesareans, but you may need to be vocal and adamant about needing your doula to accompany you.

• **Being Continuously Accompanied**

Can your support person/people stay with during all stages of surgical preparation? For some reason, many hospitals separate birthing women from their support team during the final check of the OR or during the "prep" of the mom for surgery. This can mean that the mother is alone for fifteen to thirty minutes. While the medical team talks to each other about their preparation, the woman can easily become frightened and anxious about what is ahead. She is likely to be thinking about what it will feel like as well as experiencing any emotions about the loss of the experience of natural birth. This anxiety would be much easier to deal with if she were not separated from her team.

• **Documentation of Your Baby's Birth**

Do you want photographs? Videos? Who will hold the camera?

• **Immediate Skin-to-Skin Contact**

This is becoming more common, but you may want to be prepared to insist on this.

• **Breastfeeding in the OR**

There is no reason you can't put your baby to the breast even as the surgeons finish the surgery on your abdomen. Some women prefer to just snuggle their babies during this time, but breastfeeding should be available and supported if you want to try right away and if your baby is rooting for the breast.

• **Witnessing Your Baby's Birth**

Does your hospital have clear drapes that allow you to see your baby being born (but still blocks your vision of the incision area)? If not, could they lower the drape partway so you could witness your baby's arrival into the world?

• Use of Your Arms

You can request that the anesthesiologist not tie down your arms during the surgery (the worst part for some women in the past). You can also request that IV lines be inserted in your nondominant arm, so your dominant arm is available for holding and touching your baby.

• Use of Mother's Preferred Music

• Request Medical Staff to Keep Conversation Professional

Casual talk between doctors and nurses in the OR can be disorienting to the family going through this emotionally heightened experience. It may be "all in a day's work" for the staff, but it is a major life event for you.

• Vaginal Swabs

This is a new practice and the scientific evidence is still not fully in. However, in the absence of clear scientific evidence, it is worth researching and making up your own mind about vaginal swabbing. The doctors would insert a sterile swab into your vagina and later wipe it on your baby's skin and mouth. This simulates the bacterial experience your baby would have had during a vaginal birth. These bacteria are normally the first to colonize a baby's gut and form an important part of the baby's immune system.

Your Turn

What is the essential message you would like to communicate to your birth team? What are the key areas to include? In one page or less, in positive language, put pen to paper (or fingers to keyboard) and write the first draft of your birth plan.

As you read the following chapters, you may find more ideas that you would like to include. Hone your birth plan as you read and as you advance through your pregnancy. Usually women are ready to finalize their birth plans somewhere between months five and eight of pregnancy.

Ruth Ann's Birth Preferences for the Hospital

I am planning a natural birth. I've never done this before, and I am scared, but hopeful, prepared, and determined. Please support me in this endeavor.

Beginning Labor

- I would like to begin labor naturally. If my bag of waters breaks first, I would like to wait for contractions to begin on their own.

People in the Room

- I request that no residents or students be present during my labor.

- I would like my husband and possibly my friend Susanna to be present for labor and delivery. If it is helpful to my labor, I may also like to have my sisters or other friends present.

First-Stage Labor

- I (really, really!) hope to use water during labor and delivery to ease pain.

- I am aware that pain medication is available. If I need it, I will ask for it.

- I request that the hospital staff suggest natural ways to manage pain (for instance, shower, whirlpool tub, massage, position change, walking).

Second-Stage Labor

- I would rather risk a tear than have an episiotomy.

Cesarean Section

- I strongly hope to avoid a cesarean.

- If a cesarean becomes necessary, I would like my husband to be present at all times during the operation.

- I would like to be conscious.

- I would like to hold or touch my baby immediately afterward, before an examination.

Post-Birth

- I would like to hold my baby immediately after birth.

- I would like the staff to wait until the umbilical cord stops pulsating before clamping it.

- I would like my husband to cut the umbilical cord.

- I do not want routine Pitocin postpartum.

- I would like to postpone routine newborn procedures until after I have held and breastfed my baby for the first time. I would especially like to postpone eye ointment.

- I would like all newborn procedures to take place in my presence, while I or my husband is touching the baby.

- I plan to breastfeed.

Zafira's Birth Plan

- I plan to give birth naturally with the support of my mother and sister.

- I ask for your assistance to make this day holy and reverent.

- When my baby is born, according to my religion, the first words he or she should hear are words of praise for Allah. As soon as the baby is born, please open the door for my husband so he can perform this ritual.

- I hope to stay with my baby at all times, but in the case that we are separated, please place the attached card in the baby's chart or on the bassinet. [Zafira included a handwritten card that read, "Please do not praise child without parents present." In her culture, praising a baby is considered bad luck.]

CREATING A SUPPORTIVE TEAM

Y OUR BIRTH TEAM WILL ULTIMATELY INCLUDE a great number of people. Many of these people are chosen for you by the hospital: your nurses, medical students, residents, and so on. However, you do get to shape your birth team in many important ways.

Many hospitals have a policy that only two persons, in addition to medical personnel, can attend a birth (a spouse plus a doula, for example). Increasingly, doulas report that most hospitals are not including a doula in this count. Many mothers find that this hospital rule is a handy way to "uninvite" family members: "I'm sorry," you can say to your mother, "the hospital will allow only two people to come with me." In practice, however, many hospitals are lax about enforcing the rule. I attended a birth at one hospital with this rule, but my client's tight-knit family ignored it completely. Her parents and four sisters showed up at the hospital and spent many hours actively supporting my client in labor. If hospital staff are actively enforcing the two-at-a-time policy, there is an easy way around it. Your support people can take turns in the labor room and spend the rest of the time in the hospital lounge.

Some people you may want to include on your team are

• your medical care provider (a midwife, family doctor, or obstetrician);

• your spouse or partner, if you have one;

- a professional doula;

- a good friend who is supportive of your birth choices;

- relatives such as your mother, father, or sister; and

- older siblings of your baby.

It is vitally important that all the people who take part in the birth support your birth plan. In Chapter Three, I touched on the question of whom to invite from among your family and friends. That chapter will help you decide, by examining events in your past, which individuals could be good support persons for you. In this chapter, I will also guide you in choosing professional helpers, such as a medical care provider and a professional doula.

How Many People Should Be Invited?

Most professional birth attendants recommend limiting the number of people that you invite to the birth. Michel Odent, a French physician who has passionately advocated natural birth in hospitals, believes that when a woman in labor is being observed, her energy is dissipated. In fact, if a woman's labor plateaus, he recommends leaving her alone to help labor get reestablished. Midwives often tell tales about births in which a conflict between family members interfered with the birth process. When the offending relative left the room, labor progressed more smoothly.

For a first birth, you will probably do best to invite fewer rather than more people. Choose whom to invite based on what you need, not on what will make your relatives or friends happy. Though you may feel uncomfortable inviting one sister and not another, you would feel more uncomfortable experiencing extra hours of contractions because of an unwanted observer's presence.

I urge you to follow your heart in this matter. Though many well-respected midwives and doctors believe firmly that a small number of birth attendants is ideal, I know that many women, myself included, long for what I call a community birth. At the birth of my second child, my team consisted of my husband and two doulas. At my third labor, I was attended by a robust group of ten—my midwife, two doulas, and other friends for me; a doula specifically for my husband; and my two older children and their caretakers. Everyone had an important role and added positively to my experience. As an extrovert who gets energy from other people, I would have made a mistake by inviting only a few people to my baby's birth.

Older Siblings at the Birth

In our culture, it is rare for children to attend the births of younger siblings. For some older siblings, however, attending the birth creates lifelong memories and a bond with the new family member. Even just participating in early and active labor at home, and not attending the birth at the hospital, can be a positive experience. There is no right answer to whether or how your older child should participate in your birth experience, but there are a few questions you can ask yourself to help decide:

- Is the child old enough to remember the labor or birth in the long run? (Most children under the age of five, and all those under the age of four, are unable to remember details of life experiences the way that older children do.)

- Does your older child generally need your attention when you are together?

- Can you imagine yourself grunting, groaning, or even screaming in front of your child?

- Will you feel free to do or say whatever you need in your child's presence?

- How will your child feel when seeing you in pain?

If you do decide to invite an older sibling, take care of a couple of practical matters. First, assign an adult to take care of your child during labor. Your child should feel free to leave the room at any time. Some children leave because they are bored, some because they are overwhelmed. Because you cannot predict your child's reaction, your child's babysitter should be ready to leave the birth scene when necessary.

Therefore, this babysitter should not be your primary source of emotional support (such as your partner or doula). Second, consider watching a video about birth that you have prescreened to help your child understand what is about to happen.

Your Medical Care Provider

Your caregiver's stance on natural birth will have a tremendous effect on your experience, though not because your caregiver will be with you throughout your labor. On the contrary, most obstetricians and family doctors do not attend their clients' labors, though they may occasionally check in by phone. In most cases of natural hospital birth, physicians attend only in the final hour or so. They are there when the baby is born, when the placenta arrives, and when stitches are needed. Through the rest of labor, hospital nurses generally provide most of the care. Hospital midwives tend to spend more hands-on time with their clients in labor than physicians do, but how much time a particular midwife may be present depends on factors such as how many clients she has in labor at the same time and whether a laboring woman has effective support people with her.

Even though doctors and midwives may not be present during labor, their opinions about birth shape the mother's experience, through the way they handle prenatal care and through their decisions to intervene in nature's plan. Your doctor's or midwife's opinions about how labor should begin are critical. Will your caregiver wait patiently and confidently for contractions to begin even if you are twelve days beyond your estimated due date? What if your water breaks before you feel contractions? Or will he be nervous about waiting, even though studies show that, in the absence of fever and other symptoms, it is almost always safe to wait for labor to begin on its own? (There is more information about this topic later in this chapter.) Because nurses know how individual practitioners tend to view particular situations in labor, your course of care in the hospital will most likely reflect your caregiver's style.

A thoughtful choice of caregiver goes a long way toward ensuring a good birth experience. Most women make this choice after one meeting with one member of a practice. Much more is necessary to ensure the right match. This section is designed to help you go beyond the interview to make the best choice possible.

Unfortunately, first interviews with midwives and obstetricians do not usually give you the information you need to make an informed decision. Almost all practitioners will say that they support natural birth and breastfeeding. Almost every obstetrician will say, "I do C-sections and episiotomies only when absolutely necessary." Though their words are identical, one practitioner who claims to support natural birth may have a 45-percent C-section rate, and another only a 10-percent rate. You are looking for professionals with lower-than-average intervention rates. Frank Anderson, M.D., M.P.H., an obstetrician in Michigan, comments that obstetricians may not "know what supporting natural birth really means, so they say they support it but don't really know what they are supporting."

But statistics do not tell you everything. As Anderson points out, "A maternal-fetal medicine specialist [an obstetrician with extra training in high-risk birth] may have a high C-section rate because he or she has such high-risk patients but could still be very open to natural birth."

This chapter will teach you how to find caregivers who support natural birth in action, not just words. First, I will describe your three main choices of caregiver. Knowing the different ways in which these practitioners are trained can help you hone in on the right questions to ask. Then, I will explain how to use local resources to create a list of practitioners to interview.

Types of Practitioners: Obstetricians, Family Doctors, and Midwives

The first fact to consider about the differences among these professional categories is that doctors and midwives are first and foremost people and only secondarily birth professionals. Whether a caregiver relies on heavy technological interventions or sits on her hands to let nature do most of the work depends largely on her level of trust in nature. Some obstetricians have high trust in nature, and some midwives do not. I never assume that a midwife is more natural-leaning than a physician.

Historically, the training of midwives and the training of physicians have been different. How these professionals apply their training depends on their personalities and their own life histories. In general, midwives tend to see far more natural births during their training than physicians. Physicians tend to see far more complications. Obstetricians see the most complications of all.* These three types of professionals are experts in different areas. Because of their training, midwives are experts in natural birth and in preventing complications. Family doctors are authorities on standard, medicalized hospital birth and can lean in either a more natural or a more medical direction. Finally, obstetricians are experts in handling birth complications.

Statistics from nations with better maternal and infant outcomes than ours, such as the Netherlands, and global research by affiliates of the World Health Organization show that emergency skills and technology are needed in about 10 to 15 percent of births (World Health Organization 2015; Betran et al., 2007; Davis-Floyd et al., 2009). All three kinds of caregivers are trained in handling birth emergencies. Whether you hire an obstetrician, a family doctor, or a midwife, you can be assured that if something goes wrong, your caregiver will use whatever technology and expertise are needed to ensure the best outcome (for a family doctor or a midwife, this may mean calling an obstetrician). What you cannot be assured of is that your caregiver will not use technology if you fall into the 85 percent of birthing women who do not need interventions.

For many women, the overuse of technology seems like a small price to pay to ensure a good birth outcome and avoid pain. Though scientific evidence remains on the side of judiciousness, many women are unaware of any risks to interfering in the birth process when it is going well. I remind you of this here because practitioners are not used to women with a strong commitment to natural birth.

For women with such a commitment, an important consideration is how experienced a caregiver is with natural birth. This is what you must find out! Questions about attitudes or opinions about natural birth will elicit attitudes and opinions. What you need to dig for is actual experience.

---

* Some obstetricians seek extra training in prenatal complications, such as multiple pregnancies, surgical intervention during pregnancy, or pregnancies in women with heart disease or diabetes. These maternal-fetal specialists usually manage only complicated pregnancies.

Here is a fact that may surprise you: Obstetricians may never see a single natural birth during medical training, and some may never see more than a handful in their entire careers. If an obstetrician's practice averages a 10-percent natural-birth rate, which is higher than for many, this means that 90 percent of the births the doctor attends are medically managed. Few obstetricians have been with a woman in labor from beginning to end, over the many hours often needed for progression from 1 to 10 centimeters and then pushing out the baby. Obstetricians' training focuses on the moment of delivery, surgery, and serious complications. Because of this emphasis, obstetricians may have few personal encounters with long natural labors.

When a practitioner has a low rate of natural births, I am curious about the few births that are natural. In a high-tech practice, the natural births can sometimes be mistakes. A labor-and-delivery nurse in Michigan confided to me that most of the "natural" births overseen by particular doctors at her hospital are of the super-fast, too-late-for-an-epidural variety.

Whereas medical-school students must attend a minimum number of births with interventions such as C-sections, epidurals, forceps, vacuum deliveries, and episiotomies, there is no requirement that these students attend even a single natural birth. What this means is that doctors have in-depth knowledge of how to measure a cervix and extract a baby with surgical tools, but they may have only theoretical knowledge of natural labor. If your doctor has seen few or no labors progress from start to finish without medical intervention, he compares your labor to medicalized labors, not to natural labors. Since most women, especially the first time around, have labors that last more than fourteen hours, it's important to know whether your caregiver has had natural-birth clients with long labors. It isn't helpful for your caregiver to think that birth can be all-natural only if your labor goes fast.

Midwives, by contrast, see hundreds of all-natural labors. When your labor plateaus, most midwives can easily remember other labors that have plateaued and then continued without drugs. Most obstetricians do not have this experience because most plateaus in hospitals are treated with interventions. Most midwives have attended women who have pushed for several hours. Most obstetricians would never let their clients push for hours, so they have little or no experience with this option.* Many midwives have attended women in labor from start to finish; most obstetricians have not.

Let me reemphasize, however, that training alone does not make a caregiver. Experience, too, is vital. Many factors contribute to an individual practitioner's style. Some obstetricians love natural birth. They are eager for a break from their high-risk patients and the chance to attend a beautiful, uncomplicated birth. These obstetricians may attend many high-risk women yet always do their best to use minimal technology. And some midwives, especially those who feel tenuous at hospitals that do not fully support midwifery care, may be quick to intervene so that they don't "get into trouble."

Make a List of Potential Caregivers: Talk to the People Who Know

Before you meet with any practitioners, I recommend consulting people in your community about whom to interview. Your three best sources of information are homebirth midwives, experienced local doulas, and mothers who have had positive birth experiences.

You might be surprised to see homebirth midwives on this list of resources. You are not planning a homebirth, so you may feel awkward about calling them. However, since you are not a potential client, they are your most objective source of information. Ask them which obstetricians, doctors, and hospital midwives in town have the highest rates of natural birth. A homebirth midwife will probably be able to give you several names right away. The Internet is an easy way to find homebirth midwives to call or e-mail.

Doulas who have worked for several years in your community will have observed the working style of many local practitioners. Most women who hire doulas are aiming for a natural birth in a hospital, so doulas are a gold mine of information. They know which hospitals, which

---

Obstetricians base many of their decisions and protocols on evidence from studies of birth. But many of the studies used as the evidence base for obstetrical practices, such as how long a woman can safely push, compare one intervention to another rather than to natural birth, or are confounded by the use of multiple interventions.

nurses, and which doctors are the easiest to work with and which push medical interventions the most. There may be a doula organization in town that can give you the names, phone numbers, and e-mail addresses of members. Otherwise, again, you can employ the Internet.

Finally, mothers who have given birth in your area can be an excellent source of information, although usually not as good a source as midwives and doulas. Most mothers have firsthand experience with only one or two midwifery or obstetrical practices. A new mother usually has a strong opinion about her caregiver, but she cannot objectively compare her caregiver's style with that of others. Still, when you seek out stories of moms in your area who had positive birth experiences, it's worth asking them questions about their caregivers.

Be careful about using negative stories as your guide. Most of the time it is impossible to know whether a single negative story is part of a larger pattern or an aberration. Even the best practitioners attend births that don't go the way the mother wishes. Positive stories, though, are generally a good guide. If a practitioner offered one woman consistent support for a natural birth, this practitioner may indeed have the skills and values that you are looking for.

Interview Potential Caregivers

Once you've made a list of recommended caregivers in your area, start calling them and make appointments with the most promising. Though you may be able to get some information in a quick phone conversation, you will learn much more from an in-person office visit. Here are some questions you might ask at an initial interview:

Q. *Can you tell me what kind of birth you chose for yourself [or what kind your partner chose], and what you learned from it?*

> **A.** If a midwife or physician has children and is willing to discuss their births, you will learn a lot. Caregivers bring all their personal experience, thoughts, and opinions to a birth, even if they try not to. This is not a matter of professionalism. It is human nature to learn from our own experiences. But a physician who gave birth by a C-section might still be a good match for you.

Listen for signs of her attitude about her C-section. If she jokes that she was "lucky" to miss the pain of labor, you might want to move on. But if she wishes her labor could have gone differently, she might remain on your list.

You might be surprised to learn that some hospital practitioners have given birth at home. These practitioners can be gems, professionals who trust in natural birth.

Q. *Can you tell me about the most recent natural birth you attended?*

A. If the person you are interviewing has to think hard to retrieve an example, you have just gained valuable information. If instead the practitioner smiles, sits back, and describes a recent inspiring birth, you have also gained valuable insight. If the birth described was quick, ask the caregiver to describe the last long natural labor she attended.

Q. *In your opinion, what helps women achieve natural birth? What can a woman do to prepare?*

A. Stumbling for answers here means that a practitioner does not often ponder these questions. Her focus is probably on the external and mechanical side of birth, not on the birthing woman's own emotional and physical preparation. This practitioner may believe that whether a woman has a labor that she can handle is entirely the luck of the draw.

If instead the practitioner has an immediate opinion that makes sense to you, you might be able to work together. You are looking for someone who believes that what women do in labor matters.

Q. *In your professional opinion, what are the main reasons that women who want natural births do not have them?*

A. A common, evasive answer to this question is, "Birth is unpredictable. Anything can happen. It doesn't help to get too attached to the idea of birth going a certain way." (If you have read Chapter Three, you understand that, although birth is unpredictable, it does indeed help to get attached to the idea of birth going a certain way.) This answer informs you that this practitioner is not very committed to helping women achieve a natural birth; she is more concerned that her clients learn to accept medical interventions.

But consider the comment of a very experienced family doctor in Ann Arbor. In the 1970s, he told me, when a woman said she wanted a natural birth, she came to the hospital prepared to withstand physical pain. Nowadays, he finds that women are more likely to say they want natural birth but less likely to do the necessary mental preparation. If I were interviewing him to be my caregiver, I would be encouraged that he thinks the locus of control is within the woman. I would ask follow-up questions about what kind of preparation he believes to be helpful.

Q. *What do you think birth pain means to women? What is the value of birth pain?*

A. This question will probably take many practitioners by surprise. You can easily contrast answers like, "It's not a contest. There's no medal for enduring pain" with, "I think it means something different to each woman. I'm always amazed at what women have to say after they give birth."

As you ask these questions, a caregiver may assume that you, like so many women before you, will change your mind about natural birth while you are in labor. Your doctor or midwife and your labor-and-delivery nurses are used to women who say they want a natural birth but ultimately choose pain medications. This is a key factor in the way these birth professionals will interact with you. It helps to have empathy for them. Having seen this reversal far more often than successful natural birth, they have no way of knowing that you are different.

Practitioners who often intervene in the birth process may feel attacked by your questions. They may act defensive or superior and may remind you that you are not an "expert." A defensive attitude is not what you need in a caregiver. Ideally, you want a practitioner who is open to what is right for you. As a doula, I am committed to helping women get the birth experiences they are seeking. This sometimes means helping a woman get an epidural or a C-section. My opinion about birth is not important. Supporting the birthing woman is important. If you run into a defensive caregiver (or, worse, a practitioner who goes on the attack), keep looking.

Trust Your Instincts

So far, we have focused on finding a birth professional who is able to support a natural birth. In addition to having experience, training, and skills, as well as respect for your values, your ideal practitioner must be a person whom you enjoy being around and whom you trust.

As I explained in Chapter Two, you must not only be safe during labor; you must also feel safe. This is a subjective assessment you must make according to your own history and intuition about people. Giving birth is different from having a broken leg fixed. If you do not like the doctor who is setting your leg, everything will probably turn out fine anyway. If you do not like and trust the person who is with you in labor, your body can turn the process off.

When you interview a caregiver, you will know right away whether there is good rapport. One picky client in New York City interviewed several midwives before finding a good match. The first midwife ignored her husband during their meeting and sent him out of the room for the physical exam. Another midwife chattered nonstop throughout the session. These factors influenced her final decision. She ultimately picked a caregiver who treated both her and her husband warmly and who listened as much as she spoke.

Inviting Your Birth Team on Board with the Plan

Once you've hired a caregiver, you still have work to do.

Most likely you have hired not just one practitioner but an entire practice. The average North American woman meets with two to six different caregivers during prenatal visits, knowing that any one of them might be on call the day she gives birth. You are fortunate if you find a small practice, with one to three caregivers. Scientific evidence reveals that "continuous care," which means that the same familiar person provides prenatal care and attends the birth, is ideal. (If you hire a practitioner in a solo practice, be sure you understand his plans for backup care. You need to know who will care for you if he is sick or attending a birth at a different hospital when you go into labor.)

Whether you meet with one or six different caregivers, however, one of your jobs during prenatal visits is to invite your birth team on board with your birth plan. As your pregnancy progresses and you meet with your caregiver, you will ask a lot of questions about your growing baby and your health concerns. Bringing such questions to these meetings is important. Equally important is bringing evidence of your growing excitement about natural birth. Your enthusiasm and confidence are the keys to persuading even reluctant caregivers to join you in pursuit of your worthwhile goal. In the following sections, I give you some ideas about how to share your enthusiasm.

Share Stories

For each prenatal visit, give yourself the homework assignment of bringing a new story about a natural birth. Copy stories from magazines, books, or the Internet that touch you. Once or twice in your pregnancy, share these copies with your practitioner. At the top of the story you can write a note such as "I wanted to share this beautiful birth story. I found it really inspiring." Your practitioner may or may not read the story, but it may well end up in your file. Every time you arrive for a prenatal checkup and again at the birth, your caregiver will open a file and find there a story that inspires you. This sends a strong, positive message about your birth plan. It shows that you value natural birth and also that you are doing real research about what natural birth is like. It shows that natural birth is not just a passing fashion for you.

When you do not share a paper copy of an inspiring story, tell a positive birth story instead. Say that your neighbor, for instance, recently gave birth at the same hospital that you'll be using, that she had a "lovely birth," and that she felt "so supported."

Introduce Your Birth Plan with Reverence

When my daughter began violin lessons at age seven and a half, her teacher did not just hand her a violin and a bow and let her begin playing. The teacher first taught my daughter reverence for the instrument. My daughter practiced the correct feet positions for playing or resting with the violin. She practiced holding a pen in her hand as if it were a violin bow, and she moved the pen up and down and side to side to learn how to move the bow. She even had to master latching and unlatching the case properly before she was allowed to—finally!—hold the instrument.

The reverence taught in these first lessons was a strong foundation for the years ahead. When my daughter comes home sweaty and tired from playing outdoors, and I must encourage her to wash her hands before violin practice, she may resist a bit, but deep down she has the feeling that washing her hands is worth the trouble. The act of creating beautiful music deserves her full attention, her awe and veneration. It is not a throwaway activity with little meaning.

Your baby's birth will be an awe-inspiring event that will change your life forever. Let your caregivers know how reverently you are preparing for it. Though you will ultimately share a one-page, succinct birth plan with them, you can talk about your progress all along the way. Let them know at an early prenatal appointment that you are engaged in a long process of getting to know yourself as you put together your birth plan. You can share elements of your ideal birth with them. For instance, Ruth Ann told her practitioners that she often fantasized about walking on the beach during labor. The practitioners and Ruth Ann herself knew this was not likely going to be part of her real labor, but Ruth Ann wanted to talk about what birth meant to her, not just whether there was protein in her urine.

Your caregiver may ask, "Do you have any questions?" but she is unlikely to ask, "How are you feeling about the upcoming birth? What have you been thinking about?" If she does ask, great! If she doesn't ask, bring up the topic. By sharing your thoughts, you are inviting your practitioner to see the birth holistically. Unless you volunteer to share these personal parts of your birth planning with her, she doesn't have much to go on besides blood tests and heart tones.

Sometime around month six of pregnancy, you should bring in your medical birth plan. Take care with the way you introduce it. Often, families hand over the document, the practitioner skims it and asks a few questions, and it goes in the file.

Instead, bring several copies with you, so that you and your partner can each hold one. Consider prefacing the handoff with some words about how deeply meaningful the process of imagining birth has been for you. You might say, "I'm excited to share this with you. I have learned so much from thinking about all the different aspects of what this birth could be like."

Then, I suggest that you take the lead in going through the plan. You do not need to read each line verbatim. There are probably a few areas, however, where it will be helpful to ask your practitioner directly to support you. For instance, Zafira, from Chapter Three, would probably highlight her desire that no one speak at the moment of birth until her husband has read holy words to the baby. In addition to such unique desires, there are two subjects that almost all women should address: how labor will begin and freedom to choose one's own position for giving birth.

As you will learn in greater depth in Chapter Seven, an important predictor of whether you will be able to achieve a natural birth is whether labor is allowed to begin on its own. This is essential to address in your birth plan because it is something over which you and your team have control. You will have little or no power over whether your labor plateaus at 7 centimeters or whether your baby's heart rate dips too low. So take charge of this issue that you can positively control. Talk to your practitioner about the two common scenarios in which births are induced: when a woman goes past her due date (or, in some practices, when she gets close to her due date) and when a woman's waters break before contractions begin. Specific recommendations for how to handle this second scenario begin on page 153.

Tell your practitioner that you want to concentrate on this topic because it is one of the few over which you have some control. The practitioner will understand that. Ask about her protocol for inductions. Does she induce labor when a woman reaches thirty-nine weeks' gestation? When a mother goes past her due date by a day or two? When she goes past her due date by a week? What is the longest your caregiver has waited for labor to occur naturally? If a woman's waters break, what is the practitioner's standard practice? Many caregivers and many hospitals have protocols dictating that the baby should be born within a certain number of hours after waters break, even though studies show that it is almost always safe to wait for labor to begin on its own, in the absence of fever and other symptoms. (See Chapter Eight, for a thorough discussion of this situation.)

It is all right to ask for support for your plan, with as much respect as you can, even if your caregiver follows an early induction protocol. I know of dozens of women whose doctors have made exceptions to their usual way of doing things. Without saying that the doctor is wrong, you can emphasize how important it is to you to let labor start naturally. You can say you know that artificially induced contractions often hurt more than natural contractions and you do not want to have to use pain medications. Say you know, too, that many inductions "don't work," and that in these cases, women spend hours or even days in the hospital and then are too exhausted for a natural birth. Since many of these women don't have their hearts set on a natural birth, a failed induction may not be so bad for them. But you do want a natural birth, so this would be disastrous for you!

Ask for your practitioner's support from the heart. You do not want to dispute the benefits of induction on medical grounds because unless you are a birth professional yourself, you would probably lose (if you are a birth professional, then go for it). The strength of your argument comes from what this birth means to you, which is not something the doctor can counteract with facts from a study.

A Final Note on Conversations during Prenatal Visits

Though I am advocating that you bring confidence to your prenatal visits, I do not mean that you must be entirely sure of yourself. It is natural and normal to have doubts, especially in a first pregnancy, about whether you can give birth naturally. Expressing these doubts to your caregiver is perfectly fine. But you should also express deep, unwavering confidence that giving birth naturally is worthwhile and meaningful for you, even if it is scary.

Bringing Support People with You to Prenatal Visits

Prenatal visits with obstetricians average thirteen minutes (Gottschalk & Flocke, 2005), and some midwifery practices keep appointments to half an hour. For your partner, best friend, doula, or sister to take time off from work to accompany you to such a short, mostly physical appointment can seem like a waste of time. Bring them anyway!

The presence of a support person at each prenatal checkup makes your pregnancy and birth stand out to your practitioner as something larger than a physical event. It humanizes you, the client. Your baby's birth is such an important part of your life that you are bringing parts of your life with you to these appointments. Coming along on prenatal visits also helps your partner focus on the birth and get to know your doctor or midwife. During labor, your partner will be able to communicate with your caregiver much more easily than you. Allowing this relationship to develop early is helpful.

Switching Caregivers Mid-Pregnancy

If this is your first baby, you will probably learn a lot about pregnancy and birth while you are pregnant. Your ideas about birth may change dramatically between the time of conception and the time of delivery. The doctor who was just right for you in month one may be entirely wrong for you in month seven. For this situation, the advice I got from the women I interviewed who were unhappy with their birth experiences is unequivocal: switch caregivers!

Nurse-midwife Julia Seng describes one woman who switched caregivers late in pregnancy. This woman, a cancer survivor, found that the way her obstetrician interacted with her during her pregnancy reminded her too much of her cancer treatment. When she realized that her obstetrician was not likely to change his ways, she interviewed a different care provider, a midwife. She told the midwife that she did not want to feel like a cancer patient during the birth. The midwife squeezed her hand and said, "We don't want you feeling like a patient either. We want you feeling like a strong, gutsy mom." In the end, this mother remained upright throughout active labor and gave birth wearing a football jersey from her alma mater. The shirt helped her feel like the "strong and gutsy" mom of the boy she was delivering.

You may be stuck, I know, with your current practitioner. There may be no other caregivers in your area who are accepting patients. Or your insurance may bind you to a particular practice. Or you may have a high-risk condition that limits your choices. Even in one of these situations, make sure you have really exhausted your resources. A less-than-perfect caregiver can make your birth experience less than perfect, too. Switching is worth the time, effort, and whatever social discomfort it might entail.

Women often realize, toward the end of their pregnancies, that they are serious about wanting a natural birth and that their caregiver's answers to questions are unsatisfactory. I have known dozens of women who switched caregivers at the eleventh hour. I have learned from their stories that asking for what you truly want is always worth it. Women have negotiated reduced fees or an agreement to pay over time, or both, when their insurance wouldn't cover the practitioner they wanted. Other women have found hospitals and caregivers farther from home that fit their needs better.

You may feel awkward leaving a practitioner with whom you have interacted for months. You may worry about upsetting the person. But women who stay with their doctor or midwife to avoid embarrassment often regret it. If you feel paralyzed about taking action, ask a friend or doula for help. Sometimes, just having someone we respect agree that it's a good idea to switch makes us feel like we have permission. We are not weak if we need a bit of handholding through the process. We are sensitive humans.

Whether you find the right match at the beginning or only weeks before your due date, hiring a supportive caregiver is worth it.

Childbirth-Preparation Classes

Be Smart About Online Research

In the Internet age, we have become used to researching almost anything in the privacy of our own homes. Birth is a booming Internet business. As the Internet has taken over as an information provider, attendance at childbirth-preparation classes has declined dramatically (Declercq et al., 2014).

If so many women are using the Internet to prepare for childbirth, where are women getting their information? Studies show that nearly 70 percent of childbearing women watch reality TV programs about birth. Unfortunately, watching these shows has been proven to increase women's fear. That's no surprise because the needs of a TV producer are exactly the opposite of a woman in labor. The TV producer needs to create drama and complicated plot twists; a woman in labor is served by a calm atmosphere. Since they began, reality birth shows have depicted more unusual complications, medical interventions, and heroic cesareans than occur statistically in real life. The researchers Stoll and Hall write:

> The shows overrepresented complications of pregnancy, in an attempt to increase the entertainment value of the episode, and showed doctors solving problems and saving mothers' and babies' lives. Laboring women were often depicted as helpless and childlike; they tended to be rewarded for complying with doctors' suggestions (e.g., to have an induction or a CS [cesarean]), whereas the few women who had a natural physiologic birth were characterized as out of control and in intolerable pain. (2013, p. 227).

In addition to reality shows, there are hundreds of birth videos posted to YouTube and a plethora of websites and blogs devoted to birth. Women often join an online "Due Date" discussion club through these websites, where they can ask questions and share information with other women who are at the same stage of pregnancy.

For a natural-birth-minded pregnant woman, these discussion forums can be a mixed bag. On the one hand, there is certainly great value in connecting with and sharing stories with women going through the same things. No one understands what it feels like to have to take care of a toddler while feeling nauseous all day like another mother in the same situation. On the other hand, U.S. and Canadian birth culture definitely slants toward medicalization of even the most routine aspects of pregnancy and birth. Some women find it disheartening to endure long discussion threads about epidural plans or cesareans planned for going past a due date. In particular, in the discussion forums I have participated in for research, I was shocked at the sharp turn toward talk of induction around week 37 and 38. The majority of women expressed impatience and readiness to "just be done" with pregnancy; the women who advocated waiting for babies to come on their own timeline were in the minority, perhaps because they were often ridiculed.

I think it is a great idea to join an online community during pregnancy. If you do so, I urge you to look beyond the commercial, mainstream, for-profit websites. There are wonderful Facebook groups, for example, specifically for women who are planning natural births. Two I recommend are "Natural Birth Support Group" and "Natural Hospital Birthing." Be forewarned that many groups have rules about what members can post about topics such as vaccinations and inductions. Though controversial issues can get complicated online, the exuberant, empathetic, and instant feedback from other mothers in these groups is worth that hurdle. Many local communities even have their own online groups. If you have trouble finding a natural-birth online community, ask doulas or midwives in your town. They are likely to have recommendations.

Likewise, when you seek information about pregnancy or birth online, be careful of your sources. If you are sure that you want a natural birth, you should seek out evidence-based information online as well as positive natural birth stories. Go-to resources these days include evidencebasedbirth.com and lamaze.org. Lamaze also has a blog with good information called givingbirthwithconfidence.org. Evidence-based Birth began in 2012 and has in-depth analysis of common practices, such as inducing women who go past their due dates. This website is helpful if you are the kind of woman who likes to do deep research in general or if you run into a specific situation in pregnancy that you need more information about. The Lamaze website offers information in a more synthesized way; however, if you want to know more about a topic, they offer papers that explain the science behind their recommendations.

Childbirth Classes Have a Lot to Offer You— and Your Partner

An online community is supportive, but it is *not the same* as a real community made up of people you can see and interact with. You will not give birth virtually in cyberspace. You will give birth, I hope, with supportive people in attendance. Childbirth-preparation classes are to birth what football practice is to a football game. Can you imagine a football team trying to play a big game without practice? How well will they execute their plays if they have discussed them only by e-mail?

Birthing women benefit from meeting each other in person, comparing notes and ideas, and, often, developing friendships that last beyond the time of giving birth. These are often the first people you call when you are having trouble nursing or need someone to run an errand. Good childbirth education classes create *real*, not virtual, communities.

Partners arguably benefit even more from classes than pregnant women. Most birth research and reading is done by the pregnant woman, which makes sense. However, who will be responsible for talking to doctors and nurses and communicating what a woman wants? Probably her partner. Childbirth-preparation classes are often the place where the idea of labor becomes real for partners and where, for the first time, they really, truly concentrate on learning about this life-changing event. When I teach childbirth-preparation classes, I insist that partners take all the notes, not the pregnant women. I remind them that during labor a birthing woman is not supposed to be thinking rationally; she is supposed to be deep in the work and action of her body. And guarding the intimate space of birth is really the partner's job. Partners may not know, unless they take classes, that they can do things like turn out the lights in a hospital room every time staff exits. These small details are not always intuitive, but they can make a big difference in a woman's birthing experience.

Many kinds of childbirth-preparation classes are available, but since you want a natural birth, I urge you to seek out an independent class geared toward supporting women who want physiologic birth. These can be hard to find because they may be taught by one person in your community, not an organization. For instance, in my area, we have individual Bradley, Hypnobirthing, Evidence-Based Birth, and Birthing from Within instructors who each operate independently. If you are not having luck finding local practitioners, you could try the national websites for some of these natural-birth preparation programs. Some of them have lists of certified instructors by city and state.

Insurance companies are more likely to cover hospital-based classes; however, you should be extremely cautious if you choose this route. Most hospital-run classes do not emphasize ways to prepare for natural birth. And you would feel lonely as the only one in a class of ten who was planning to go natural. There are some exceptions to this rule. Some hospitals, for example, hire Lamaze instructors. Lamaze is an organization that many think of primarily as teaching "breathing techniques" for labor; however, in the last decades, Lamaze has become much, much more than that. Today, Lamaze instructors are well-trained in supporting women who are planning natural births.

You can also ask a local midwife or doula to recommend classes geared toward natural birth. You need information about different positions to try during labor and visualizations that can help, and you need hands-on practice with your partner. Tips on how to talk to hospital staff in your particular hospital can be especially useful. Helpful classes show videos of beautiful, inspiring, natural births. Ideally, your class will be taught by someone who has given birth naturally and loves to help other women achieve natural birth.

Like prenatal visits, childbirth-preparation classes can be a special time-out from regular life to concentrate on the miracle of what you are doing and what you are about to do. My husband and I took a wonderful series of classes in Manhattan before our first baby's birth. Afterward, we thought we knew everything, so we did not take classes the second time around. But because we had changed and grown in the intervening years, our ideas about birth had changed, too. So, when I was pregnant with my third baby, we opted for a series of seven classes. We used this time to connect with each other and prepare for our third baby. Even though we didn't need lectures on the stages of birth, we found that we *did* need the opportunity to think through what this birth meant for us and for our two older children and how we wanted to make it like or different from our previous experiences.

Doulas

Doulas are professional labor companions. The word *doula* comes from Greek and is usually translated as "a woman who serves." In the United States and Canada today, a doula is a professional who helps women during pregnancy or labor (a birth doula) or in the first weeks after a baby is born (a postpartum doula). Though women have been helping other women give birth and take care of infants since our ancient foremothers started walking upright (and perhaps even before that!), the profession of being a doula is still quite young. The first organization in North America to train and certify doulas began operating only in 1992.

Women who give birth with doulas are usually dumbfounded to learn that most women do not. "I just don't understand it," says Wendy, the mother of two preschoolers. "Having a doula is just so great. Why wouldn't everyone want one?" Only 6 percent of women in the United States and Canada hire doulas.

As a doula myself, I know that the main obstacle to hiring a doula is ignorance. Most people have never heard of doulas or only vaguely know what they do. But among people who have heard of them, there are usually two obstacles to hiring a doula: money and a partner who feels slighted at the idea.

Are doulas worth the money? Do they usurp the role of others at the birth? Let's look at both these issues.

Doulas' fees range considerably, from around $300 to $3,000 or more. Fees in urban areas are at the high end of this scale. In most areas, though, a wonderful doula can be found in the $700 to $1,200 range. In general, the more experienced a doula is, the more she is likely to charge. Is a doula worth this money?

There are some women who give birth quickly, easily, confidently, and with supportive hospital staff who do not offer unnecessary interventions. Such women will benefit from having a doula mostly at the emotional, psychological level. They may not really "need" a doula to bring lots of tools and ideas for labor or decision-making support.

The catch is that you can't predict any of those factors. You just don't know anything about your baby's birth ahead of time. You don't know how fast your birth will be; whether complications will arise; how well you will handle the pain and sensations of *this* particular labor; or who your nurse or caregiver will be. Virtually all hospital nurses, midwives, and doctors have scheduled shifts, so women are attended by whomever is on call. If any one of these factors is not ideal, you would probably benefit from having a doula by your side.

Some budget-conscious families look at doulas as too expensive. It might surprise them to hear that even budget guru Suze Orman, who ruthlessly advises families to live within their means by cutting things that are "wants" instead of "needs," sees doulas as a necessity for birthing women. Why? Because of the proven benefits of having a doula. Like car insurance, you may not need it every day, but when you do need it, you probably really, really need it and are glad you have it. Car insurance is worth the money, even if you never end up filing a claim. Likewise, a doula is a good investment, even if you end up having a short, easy labor. You just never know ahead of time what is going to happen and you can't hire a doula thirty-six hours into labor when your doctor suggests breaking your bag of waters.

Scientific studies have shown that women have shorter labors with fewer interventions when female helpers are present. After several studies confirmed this finding, John Kennell and Marshall and Phyllis Klaus observed, in *The Doula Book* (Klaus et al., 2002), "If doulas were a drug, it would be unethical not to use it." Resources that can tell you much more about doulas include the DONA International website at www.dona.org, the Birth Arts International website at www.birtharts.org, and the book *Birth Ambassadors* by Christine Morton and Elayne Clift.

Do doulas take over the partner's role as emotional support during labor? I think here, the case is even more unequivocal. Doulas support partners, not take over for them. Most partners have never seen a woman give birth before the birth of their own children, so it makes sense they are not equipped with the tools and skills most natural labors demand.

They know how to love their partner; they do not know how to nudge a posterior baby to change position.

Every doula training organization that I know of explicitly trains their doulas to support the whole family, not just the birthing woman. Doulas learn how to step in when a woman is struggling with contractions, to offer suggestions, find a position that helps, or try hands-on techniques like back pressure; however, once it is clear what works best, doulas often hand over the reins to partners. In my own case, in early labor, my husband tried to massage my shoulders. I brushed him off with (an admittedly not-very-nice), "Don't touch me!" When my doula arrived, I was in active labor. She, too, tried to massage me and I also told her, "No." But, she didn't give up immediately and tried a feathery touch on my upper back called "effleurage." It felt heavenly! As soon as he knew what to do, my husband was able to take over.

You do not have to take my word for it. You can contact the real experts about this: partners who have been supported by doulas. If you are wondering whether your partner would feel shut out or excluded by a doula's presence, the best way to discover if this is true (especially about a particular doula) is to talk to families in your area who have given birth with the doula you are considering hiring.

Here are stories that exemplify why I think hiring a doula is almost always a smart move:

A doula reminds you of what you really want. Your doula is your firm anchor in your belief that you can trust your body and that your desires for the birth are important. Hospital protocols are not designed to take your personal desires into account. Doulas help you assert yourself.

Allison gave birth at a hospital in Chicago. She went to the hospital when her waters broke. She writes,

> They confirmed that my water was leaking, and so the resident and all the other staff recommended I admit myself and get started on Pitocin and an IV antibiotic immediately. I was shocked and scared. I called our doula from the examining room, crying, "What should I do?" I had told the staff I would admit myself but I was not sure that was what I wanted. Our doula coached me back to my senses and reminded me of

*my wants. I turned and told Keith [her husband] and the staff that I
wanted to go home for a while. They paged our doctor to tell him. He
said, "Fine; when will you return?" I said, "In less than five hours."*

Allison's husband felt just as intimidated by the staff's impetus to admit
her. If they had not had a doula to call, Allison would likely have been
admitted into the hospital hours before contractions began. In such cases,
the woman is often hooked up to intravenous Pitocin and antibiotics right
away. Allison and her husband had never faced this scenario before, but
Allison's doula probably had. With the doula's help, Allison was able to
refocus on her goals for the birth and gain a few precious hours of peaceful preparation before being admitted to the hospital.

A doula can relieve your partner in a long labor. Jen and
Carlos, who had a baby at a hospital in Michigan, had supportive midwives who let Jen labor for two days and two nights without threatening
to give drugs. The couple's doula, Joy, helped them figure out that labor
pain was significantly more manageable when someone squeezed Jen's
hips together during her contractions. For forty-eight hours, Joy and
Carlos took turns squeezing Jen's hips for virtually every contraction.
During the second night, Joy called in a backup doula, who stayed about
five hours, letting Joy and Carlos get much-needed rest.

Jen was so impressed with the level of care she received from her doulas
that she later decided to become a doula herself. She is convinced that
without Joy and her backup doula, she and Carlos would have been forced
to ask for pain-relieving medication. Carlos could not have squeezed her
hips or given back pressure for forty-eight hours without help. The hospital's busy nurses and midwives could not possibly have done what her
doulas did to make the pain manageable over so many hours.

In my experience as a doula, hip squeezes and back pressure are key
labor tools for about 60 to 75 percent of women. This is a demanding
situation for partners. Having two people makes it much more manageable for everyone.

A doula is not scared of your pain. Seeing a loved one in great
pain can be torture. Though your partner cannot share your physical
pain, witnessing you in anguish may cause great emotional pain.

Imagine how it might tear at your partner's heart to hear you say, "Help me! Help me, please!"

Doulas, being human, also have a natural desire to relieve a mother's birthing pain. But they have something that most birth partners do not have: perspective on birth pain. An experienced doula has seen dozens or even hundreds of women emerge victoriously on the other side of labor. She knows that the pangs of labor are worth enduring in the end, no matter how awful they seem in the moment. She can concentrate her energy on helping in the here and now, fully confident that each contraction is useful. This is much harder for even the most supportive partner to do.

Your doula supports your partner. When women ask their partners to be their primary labor coaches, they may be slighting the experience of becoming a new parent. Remember that this is a meaningful day for your partner, too! As you become a mother, your partner is also being transformed into a parent. Partners deserve enough support to allow them to attend to their *own* feelings, including their own feelings of fear. Having to reassure the mother that all is going well and that she is safe during labor, while feeling just as frightened by what is happening, can be an unfair burden.

Emiliano remembers a doula offering him practical help that made a lasting impression. His wife was holding on to his hands and wanted him to breathe with her during difficult contractions. He couldn't imagine leaving her side to eat a meal, but after many hours of supporting her labor, he was famished. He remembers their doula feeding him an entire sandwich, a bowl of soup, and an energy bar, "discreetly, in between contractions, when Violetta's eyes were closed and both my hands were occupied." He says he felt nurtured by her willingness to do whatever was needed to support him.

Tricia, mother to a nine-month-old, recalls that her husband was queasy throughout her labor and had to stand against a wall for support during the pushing phase. Her strength came from her father and her doula, who stayed by her side.

A new father in New York recalls, "I spent eight hours thinking we were just minutes away from having a baby. It all felt like an emergency. Thank God Lisa [their doula] was there to calm us all down."

As a doula, I have pulled aside many new fathers or lesbian partners to ask them how they are feeling. Often, they are scared and worried, either about a complication that has arisen or about the mother's ability to go on. Even a few seconds' acknowledgment of their feelings can transform the experience for them. Afterward, they can usually return to the scene more confident and able to support the laboring woman.

As a dad in Toronto once told me, "I held her hand through the whole thing, but you held her birth plan in place." Note that I never stepped in to speak to the staff for this couple, but I did ask them twice if they wanted time to think about suggested interventions. That time allowed them to make conscious, not reactive, choices.

A doula focuses on you, even when everyone else is focused on the baby. The actual birth can bring a few minutes of panic if the baby does not breathe right away. A baby who needs help in the first few minutes may be whisked straight from the mother's body to a crib across the room. The medical professionals are all busy with the baby or the delivery of the placenta. A doula can really help in such terrifying moments. She can bring Mom observations of the baby, such as, "Your baby's eyes are wide open and looking at the ceiling." Or she can remind staff to do their work on the far side of the crib, so the mother's line of vision to the baby is clear.

A doula comes to your home after the birth. Most doulas visit their clients once or twice after the birth. In the first days, leaving the house with the infant is a strenuous chore, so having someone come to your house is an advantage. In the postpartum period, I have helped out in just about every way imaginable, from carrying on long conversations about how the birth went to doing laundry to running out for diapers.

If breastfeeding is not going well, we will usually spend a long time working on it. I have found it nearly impossible to abandon a new mother who is struggling with breastfeeding, and most doulas I know have said the same. We will refer new mothers to lactation consultants, but we will also provide hands-on help beyond the one or two visits the mom has paid for, if she needs this extra assistance. Since no one can predict breastfeeding problems, having a doula is like a backup plan in case breastfeeding does not come easily. Moms who struggle with

Woman to Woman, by Aminata Maraesa, is a twenty-six-minute video about doulas. Students, professors, and members of public libraries can stream this video for free at: www.kanopystreaming.com/product/woman-woman

breastfeeding not only need expert breastfeeding help; they often need more help than usual with things like housekeeping and meals. (Whether or not you hire a birth doula, you might consider hiring a postpartum doula to help out in this way.) I've also run interference with well-meaning relatives who may not be up-to-date on the science of breastfeeding. Doulas are like private social workers who make sure the new mother is mothered.

What you will get for your outlay of cash is a package that includes not only help at your labor and delivery but probably several prenatal and postpartum visits as well. A doula who has attended many women during birth brings with her a strong confidence in your ability to birth your baby. She does not answer to a hospital review board or an insurance company. She answers to you. So her entire objective is to help you achieve the birth you want.

Your Team

Taking charge of creating a positive birth team is a vital step in preparation for a natural birth. Shop carefully for the caregiver whose birth experience and vision match yours as closely as possible. Think about whether hiring a doula would enhance your birth experience. Finally, through the process of envisioning this birth and writing your birth plan (see Chapter Three), gain confidence in what natural birth means to you. Share your vision with your team so they can fully support you.

CHAPTER 5

EXTRA SUPPORT FOR SPECIAL CIRCUMSTANCES

PREVIOUS CHAPTERS HAVE FOCUSED ON the wonders and excitement of birth and preparing a birth plan. I've explained how the hormones associated with feelings of fear can derail labor. For women with uncomplicated pregnancies, defusing anxiety and visualizing a positive birth experience may be easier than for pregnant women who face special circumstances. This chapter explores three of the most common sets of circumstances that might complicate a normal pregnancy. They are giving birth to twins, giving birth after a previous cesarean section (vaginal birth after cesarean, or VBAC), and giving birth after surviving trauma.

If you fall into any of these categories, know that achieving a natural birth is possible. For women who are giving birth after surviving trauma or after a previous cesarean, achieving a natural birth can also be tremendously healing. You will probably need more support than women without your challenges. You deserve to be surrounded by birth professionals who bolster your confidence, not tear it down. Even more than other women, you may need to slow down during pregnancy and take the time to do birth-related research and to explore your emotions. Like all women, you cannot control all of what will happen during your birth, but you can write a birth plan, choose your caregivers wisely, and keep your mind and body well tuned through healthful eating, exercise, and the cultivation of a peaceful attitude toward giving birth. This chapter is devoted to helping mothers in special circumstances ward off anxieties and approach labor and birth with confidence.

Twin Birth

In most of the world, twins are born vaginally unless there is a complication that requires surgery. However, if you are pregnant with twins you probably already know that most twins in North America are born by cesarean section. What mothers of twins need most at their delivery is a practitioner experienced with the vaginal birth of twins, but the trend toward C-sections means that there are fewer and fewer doctors and midwives who gain this experience. Still, every day determined mothers of twins manage to give birth vaginally and without pharmaceutical drugs, and chances are you can, too. You will need extra support during pregnancy to aid you in making your dream a reality.

Since twins are commonly delivered by planned C-section, few nurses, midwives, and doctors have had the chance to attend more than a handful of natural, vaginal twin births. Many practitioners, assuming that multiples are best delivered surgically, pressure parents of twins to agree. The rarity of your desire for natural birth may make your life more difficult, but it may also work to your advantage. Once your hospital team is convinced that you really mean to give birth naturally, they may be secretly or even openly excited to participate. After attending my first such birth as a doula, I celebrated with the whole team. The attending obstetrician treated us to champagne.

There are genuine reasons for some mothers of twins to plan cesareans. For example, when twins share a single amniotic sac (as happens in about 1 percent of twin pregnancies), they have better chances of a good outcome if they are born surgically. But most concerns about vaginal delivery of twins are about position. Singletons usually "present" either head-down or buttocks-down (breech) at birth. A baby who presents sideways cannot be born vaginally unless she turns. Gravity works sufficiently well on singletons to ensure that they rarely lie sideways. In the case of twins, however, the larger number of body parts that can intertwine and the different sizes of the babies mean that gravity cannot do its job as effectively. Twins present in a wider variety of positions at the end of pregnancy than singletons do.

Caregivers are most optimistic about the vaginal birth of twins when they can see both babies head-down on an ultrasound scan. This happens about 40 percent of the time. The next-best situation is when the first twin is head-down and the second twin is buttocks-down, which occurs with about 25 percent of twins. Most of the time, when the second twin is in a breech position, vaginal delivery is possible. A breech presentation can sometimes make vaginal delivery unadvisable, but this is a matter of experience and opinion, not always scientific fact, and often cannot be determined ahead of time. For instance, if the breech baby shifts position after the first twin is delivered, so that her head turns upward or her foot drops below her buttocks, a vaginal birth becomes riskier. If one twin is lying sideways (which happens in about 10 percent of cases), there is a good chance she will turn into a position for delivery after the first twin is born or that the attending physician can manually turn her (Bowers, 2001). So, in any of these situations, a vaginal birth may be possible.

Other positions, such as the first twin in a side-lying or foot-first breech position, will generally result in a cesarean section. But you have a greater than 75-percent chance that your babies will present in a position favorable for vaginal delivery. Those are pretty terrific odds. If at birth your babies are in an unfavorable position, you may have to mourn the dream of a vaginal birth. But remember that mothers of singletons, too, may discover at the last hour that a vaginal birth is inadvisable. With two babies as with one, women are better off planning for a natural birth than taking a wait-and-see attitude.

If you have given birth vaginally already, your caregiver is probably going to be more comfortable with the idea of a vaginal twin birth. In obstetrical parlance, your pelvis is "proven" large enough to birth a baby. But whether you have given birth already or not, finding a caregiver who will support your natural birth plan is important. Hospital protocols prevent most hospital-based midwives from attending twin births, and even family doctors will probably tell you that you need an obstetrician. Obstetricians vary greatly in their attitudes and practices. If there is a choice of obstetricians in your area, I advise you to shop around for the one who is most natural-birth-friendly.

Mothers who have given birth naturally to twins advise women who are pregnant with two babies to engage the services of a doula early in pregnancy. Most caregivers consider a natural, vaginal birth of twins as an oddity, and even childbirth-preparation classes for parents of multiples often implicitly teach that, as one mother put it, "a multiple birth is purely a medical issue and that there isn't much the mother herself can do to facilitate it. Our class really focused on medical intervention issues, and we hardly did any natural-childbirth discussion or breathing practice."

So couples expecting twins are often grateful for the reassurance of a doula, like the one who reminded Elizabeth, over and over, that "giving birth to twins is perfectly normal." Because she was pregnant with twins, Elizabeth could not find any midwives in her area who were willing to take her as a client, so she ended up with an obstetrician who specializes in multiples. "I liked him because he was an expert," said Elizabeth, "but I felt intimidated by his assumption that I was going to end up in the operating room. I called my doula after every prenatal visit, and her confidence and trust in the birth process made me feel better."

"Don't forget to talk to other mothers who have done it," suggests Annalise. She found supportive resources on the Internet and chatted with mothers of twins across the globe before giving birth herself. "I just didn't allow any bad stories in," she says. "I sought out all the good twin birth stories I could find. There are lots out there." In Annalise's case, her first twin was head-down and the second twin was a frank breech (with buttocks down, feet up). "My OB thought I should plan on an epidural because he didn't like to deliver breeches vaginally," Annalise says. He believed that a C-section was so likely that it was better to have the epidural in place for anesthesia rather than waste time when they (inevitably) decided to do the surgery. But Annalise brought in so many stories of successful vaginal births of twins that her obstetrician eventually agreed to forgo the epidural.

Other mothers of twins have experienced the same pressure to plan for a just-in-case epidural. For example, Jacinta describes herself as a "home-water-birth-type mama" who felt unsupported in her desire for a natural birth. As a first-time mother, she wasn't well connected with other mothers who had given birth naturally, even to singletons. "I didn't know anyone with twins who had [given birth naturally], and most had had C-sections." Her obstetrician suggested that she plan to have an epidural. That way, he said, Jacinta could avoid undergoing general anesthesia in the case of an emergency cesarean. Though this is a common concern for obstetricians and expectant mothers, in reality, only a tiny percentage of women undergo general anesthesia for emergency cesareans in the United States. Usually there is enough time for a last-minute epidural.

Though Jacinta acquiesced to the obstetrician's suggestion at a prenatal visit, her heart was not in this decision. In labor, she kept putting off the epidural, hoping to wait as long as possible. As I describe in Chapter Eight, delay is one of the most successful techniques for mothers who are hoping to avoid medical procedures. Jacinta explains, "I postponed the epidural despite my labor nurse encouraging me to get one. I wouldn't consent, 'just yet.' Note that I am stubborn! Then, when it seemed about the right time to think about an epidural, the doctor came to check me and said, 'Oh, my God, she's complete!' So I had the babies about ten minutes later, with no anesthesiologist anywhere to be found, with one doctor delivering the first baby and another running in to grab the second."

Jackie, a mother of twins in Nebraska, says that the delivery of her twins was by far the easiest of her three birth experiences. She points out that twins tend to be much smaller than singletons, so her body did not have to do quite so much work to open and stretch. She found that her active labor was significantly shorter (two hours instead of ten and six for her first two babies' births), and that the pushing was much easier. Her first two babies were each over 9 pounds (4 kg); her twins were 6 pounds, 8 ounces (2.9 kg) and 5 pounds, 15 ounces (2.7 kg). This mother did not discover until her third trimester that she was carrying twins, and she was later glad about that. Any worrying about labor that she might have done early in pregnancy would have been for naught.

Another mother of twins, Gerta, also writes that her babies came quickly, probably because they were each smaller than a full-term single-ton would have been. "I think I was somewhat less focused on the pain than the scene of people running in and out of the room looking for a doctor to deliver my daughter. The one who did, left, and a new one came in for my son (I had never met either of them). My son arrived about fifteen minutes later. He was so much smaller that his delivery was really easy. The second doctor said, 'Why don't you try pushing again?' which seemed odd because I really didn't feel any need to push. But I pushed a few times, and out popped my son."

Stories like these make the birth of twins appear, if anything, easier than the birth of singletons and contrast sharply with the prevailing cultural attitudes toward twin births. In pregnancy, we are expected to fret about various possible undesirable outcomes and to prepare for the worst, and this seems especially true when it comes to delivering twins. There are higher risks of prematurity for twins, and twins do require cesarean delivery more frequently than singletons. But focusing on these risks, which still represent the minority of twin births, can prevent you from doing what is necessary to prepare for a successful natural birth.

Nothing will be gained by worrying. By focusing your thoughts and preparations on a successful vaginal delivery and reaching out for extra support to realize this vision, you have the best chance of giving birth the way you want.

Vaginal Birth after a Cesarean Section (VBAC)

If you are seeking a VBAC, you are likely facing enormous pressure to schedule a repeat cesarean. More than other pregnant women, you have to find deep inner strength and conviction to swim against the tide.

In my work as a doula, VBAC clients are my absolute favorites. It is magnificent to witness any woman discovering new depths to her strength and to see a new human being take a first breath. But it is heartwarming when a woman who has been convinced from a previous C-section that she lacks those depths then finds them.

There are five areas in which women with a history of cesarean must do homework. The first is finding hope in others' stories, some golden ring to hold on to in the midst of anxiety. The second is researching the cause of the past C-section. You may not be able to learn for certain whether your C-section was absolutely necessary, but you should reach an educated opinion. Third, you must explore your feelings about the decision to have a C-section. Fourth, if the surgery was traumatic, you must make concrete plans to ensure that if a repeat C-section becomes necessary, the experience will be as positive as possible. Finally, you must find a caregiver who is willing to avoid using drugs that induce or speed up labor. The best source that I know of online for much of the research you are likely to do is vbacfacts.com, a website run by Jen Kamel, herself a VBAC mom.

Surround Yourself with Positive VBAC Stories

You need something to believe in and to think about besides your own past birth experience. Surround yourself with successful stories. Read books about VBAC. Find women in your area who have given birth vaginally after cesareans and hear their stories. View yourself as a journalist or an anthropologist. Sit with a cup of tea and bring a long list of questions. Ask them everything!

Become an Expert on Your C-Section

Become as knowledgeable as you can about your past C-section. It's helpful to find intellectual and emotional clarity before going into a new birth experience. These are two different tasks. Intellectual clarity demands research.

You probably know what circumstances led to your C-section. I recommend that you learn everything you can about your particular situation, including whether the surgery was absolutely necessary. If it would help you or your practitioner, obtain copies of your hospital records. (You can get them directly from the hospital records department, possibly for a fee, so there is no need to ask your former practitioner for them.)

Currently, the U.S. cesarean rate is 32 percent of all births, a figure that is unnaturally high. By considering scientific studies and historical trends, we can estimate that about one-third of C-sections performed in North America are truly life-saving and that the majority are not.[*] You may know absolutely which category your cesarean fits into, or it may be impossible to

---

[*] *Studies confirm earlier World Health Organization recommendations that outcomes for mothers and babies are best when cesarean-section rates are no higher than 15 percent (Althabe & Belizan, 2006). Among healthy mothers who deliver healthy babies at term, the safety of mothers and children is uncompromised when the cesarean rate is as low as 4 percent (Johnson & Daviss 2005; Rooks et al., 1989).*

ever know. Many women avoid trying to find out yet harbor intense fear that the events leading to the first surgery will repeat themselves. Indeed, some situations are more likely to repeat themselves than others.

Reopening these wounds can be painful. Your caregivers certainly believed that a C-section was the right decision. And it was the right decision, for them. Yet it may not have been the right decision for you. It's OK if there is discrepancy. What is right for one person is not always right for another. Getting the facts will help you. With the facts, you can work on your feelings. You can also be more vocal about making sure that your caregivers, this time around, have values similar to yours.

Although some reasons for surgical birth—such as placenta previa (when the placenta obstructs part of the cervical opening) or a baby who is lying across the womb—are unequivocal, the most common reasons for cesarean sections in North America are more ambiguous. If your C-section occurred because of "failure to progress," a large baby relative to your pelvis (a condition called cephalopelvic disproportion, or CPD), or because you had a fever during a long labor, you will probably not be able to judge whether the situation was truly so serious as to warrant an emergency C-section (any C-section that is performed after labor begins is called an emergency C-section*). After your VBAC, you may be able to look back on the C-section with more knowledge—for instance, with the knowledge that you have long labors, not fruitless labors, or that your pelvis can, indeed, open to birth a baby.

If your cesarean was planned, your work may be easier. A diagnosis that your placenta was in the way of the baby, an active case of herpes, or a transverse or breech presentation may have made your case very clear. You may fear that the problem will repeat itself, but you will likely know for certain before you give birth. You can prepare for labor with your full heart, without second-guessing your body's ability to labor well. You can approach your first experience of labor with the joy and confidence as well as the trepidation of a first-time birthing woman. You have less reason to fear that your labor will not end in a vaginal delivery.

An emergency C-section is different from a "crash" or "stat" C-section, which is performed as fast as possible, often with general anesthesia instead of an epidural, because the doctors believe the life of the mother or baby is in imminent danger.

Possible Reasons for a C-Section

- The placenta attaches to the uterus in such a way that vaginal delivery is impossible.

- The baby's heart rate indicates severe distress.

- The baby's body has an abnormality that makes it difficult to be born.

- The baby's position makes vaginal birth impossible (for instance, the baby is lying crosswise).

- The baby's head is too large to fit through the mother's pelvis.

- There are twins (sometimes).

- There are triplets or more multiples.

- The mother's body has structural abnormalities that prevent vaginal birth.

- The mother has an active genital herpes infection.

- The baby has heart problems.

- The mother develops complications of high blood pressure (such as preeclampsia) that necessitate the immediate birth of the baby.

- Labor is prolonged.

- The umbilical cord slips beneath the baby or into or through the cervix.

- The mother has had a previous C-section with a vertical incision, which increases the risk that the uterine scar might separate.

But if you had a cesarean section after experiencing some labor, you may feel robbed of confidence and trust in your body. You may feel like a failure. The thought of mustering the courage to labor again may be exhausting, and the thought of yet again experiencing an unplanned surgery may be devastating. With such a heavy load of feelings, is it any wonder that when obstetricians suggest a repeat surgery, so many women agree? Just by reading this chapter, however, you are exhibiting courage. Facing the unknown of labor the first time requires bravery. But a first-time mountain climber has the advantage of innocence. How much more heroic to face a mountain the second time, with all the knowledge of your first attempt?

Two reasons for emergency C-sections, "failure to progress" and cephalopelvic disproportion, deserve detailed attention.

If "Failure to Progress" Was the Reason for Your C-Section

If your C-section followed "failure to progress," you are probably acutely aware of exactly how far you got in labor and how long it took to get there. You may remember a number, as in "I got stuck at 7 [centimeters]." Moving past that point in labor is the real trick for VBAC success. Because your partner may harbor the same fears based on the same experience, it may be crucial to have a new support person with you who can help you—and your partner—jump this all-important hurdle.

A birth story by a famous birth activist is instructive here. In 2001, I had the pleasure of taking a train ride with anthropologist and author Robbie Davis-Floyd. On our journey she told me about her two children's births. After her first labor ended in a C-section for "failure to progress," she was certain that the problem was not her body but her caregivers' lack of patience. She believed that the second time around she would again face a long labor. Her intuition even told her that it would take three days. This time she found midwives who were willing to wait through a long labor without calling it a failure.

In the book *Having a Baby: Mothers Tell Their Stories* (Bernstein, 1993), Davis-Floyd describes the vaginal birth of her son in great detail. At one point, she found herself shaking with fear. Her friend created a spontaneous ritual "to release me from this paralyzing fear that I wouldn't make it and would end up in the hospital with another C-section." All those present spoke of their fears and then symbolically threw them into a candle flame to release them. Robbie had fears to burn, and so did her husband. After the ritual, "I suddenly realized that the hour when the cesarean had happened, four years ago, was long past, and that I had finally entered completely uncharted territory. I was free! The past pattern no longer had the power to map itself onto my present experience!

My relief was overwhelming" (p. 187). After three days of labor, she gave birth naturally to a healthy baby.

Davis-Floyd had carefully planned this second birth. She had made sure there was a tub in which she could immerse herself during labor. She had chosen midwives who agreed to be patient during a long labor. She had invited a friend whose sole purpose was to "direct the energies" of the birth. This describes very well the role of a doula. The presence of a calm, stoical, accepting person whose job has nothing to do with measuring heartbeats or temperatures is needed even more at a VBAC than at most births. The mother needs a guide as she faces her own feelings. Hospital personnel are not always comfortable, experienced, or trained in helping women in this situation. Think through carefully what—and whom!—you will need for an optimal birth experience.

Many women diagnosed with "failure to progress" also experience a host of "failed" medical interventions. Before deciding to do surgery, most caregivers will try many technological interventions, such as breaking the bag of waters, using Pitocin, inserting an epidural, hooking the baby up to an internal fetal monitor, or using forceps. When these technologies fail or the baby cannot tolerate these interventions well, the caregiver will suggest a cesarean. If dilation remains the same for more than an hour or two in the hospital, these interventions are routine. If this was your experience before your C-section, make sure to read Chapter Ten for tips on getting across a labor plateau naturally.

Avoiding interventions to augment labor is important because these interventions in and of themselves often lead down the path toward a cesarean section. The most common scenario is that a woman experiences a plateau and feels discouraged, so her caregivers decide to augment her contractions with Pitocin. Pitocin can cause abnormally painful contractions. Because it is administered intravenously, it requires a woman to lie in bed. Fetal monitoring is also required. If the Pitocin does not speed things up, caregivers often recommend breaking the bag of waters. This, too, can cause labor to feel more painful. It also puts the woman on the clock (see Chapter Seven for more details). The combination of extra-painful contractions and lost mobility can quickly lead a woman to request an epidural. An epidural plus the loss of mobility can slow labor, and it can also create a fever. No one knows why epidurals cause fevers, but repeated studies have shown they often do (Sharpe & Arendt, 2017; Lieberman et al., 1997; Goetzl et al., 2004). Because these fevers tend to get worse the longer the woman receives the epidural, and because there is no way to know during labor whether the fever is caused by the epidural or an infection, a woman who develops a fever in this situation can easily end up with an unnecessary cesarean.*

Equally important as these physical issues, submitting to an intravenous drip, an artificial rupture of the bag of waters, or an epidural has the psychological effect of making a woman feel that other people are in charge of her labor. It becomes easier for her to imagine and agree to a C-section, the ultimate manifestation that other people are in control of birth.

If you remain active and mobile, you may have a long, exhausting labor, but you will remain in charge of your labor, and you will not end up with a C-section from an epidural-caused fever.

If Cephalopelvic Disproportion or "Large Baby" Was the Reason for Your C-Section

Thousands of North American women hear during labor that they cannot deliver their babies vaginally because the baby is too large or the pelvis is too small. These women often feel defeated and betrayed by their own bodies. The second time around they may wish to have a VBAC but may harbor deep fears about the ability of their bodies to birth a baby.

A tiny percentage of women truly are born with pelvic bones that will never allow a baby to pass through. A diagnosis of CPD can feel tragic, but if a woman is certain that the diagnosis is correct, she can accept a C-section in a different way from a woman whose diagnosis is uncertain. If you have ever heard that your pelvis might be too small to birth a baby, please get a second, third, and even fourth opinion, from various obstetricians and midwives. It's important to find out whether your small pelvis is supposition or your caregiver is diagnosing a true bone condition.

---

* One study shows that nearly 15 percent of laboring women receiving an epidural develop a fever of higher than 100.4°F (38°C), whereas only 1 percent of women laboring without an epidural do so. "Without epidural, the rate of fever remained low regardless of length of labor; with epidural, the rate of fever increased from 7 percent for labors less than six hours to 36 percent for labors greater than eighteen hours [emphasis mine]" (Lieberman et al., 1997).

Deformed pelvic bones were much more common in the 1700s, when our foremothers suffered from vitamin deficiencies. Most North American girls today get enough calcium and vitamin D to prevent rickets, the most common cause of pelvic bone deformity, so it is now extremely rare to find a pelvis that is not able to birth a baby.

A diagnosis of CPD is usually nothing more than guesswork. No one knows exactly how much your baby's head can change shape to fit your pelvis or how far your pelvis can open with the hormones of labor and with optimal positioning. Squatting, for instance, provides about 10 percent more space for the baby than the semi-reclining position.

A diagnosis of CPD during labor could have little to do with your pelvis or the baby's weight. It could have to do more with the baby's position, which has a dramatic influence on the second stage of labor. If your baby was born by C-section after a diagnosis of CPD, you will probably not know whether your baby's head was slightly tilted in the birth canal or the baby had an upraised arm. When a baby's head is not applied directly and evenly to a woman's cervix, labor can be extremely slow. The baby's head does a good portion of the work during labor, and if the head is even slightly tilted, labor can take a long time.

Violetta pushed for four and a half hours with her first baby (she describes the experience in Chapter Thirteen). In many hospitals, that much pushing time could lead to a cesarean section or instrumental delivery (depending on the hospital, two or three hours is often considered the maximum amount of time for a "normal" second stage). When Violetta's baby arrived, "he had one arm curled around the front of his body, the other arm above his chin up by his head, and he twirled out of me like a dancer." That hand by his chin probably made the descent through the birth canal quite a bit longer than it might otherwise have been. But, like millions of women before her, with patience and determination, Violetta was able to naturally deliver a baby with a hand by his head.

The idea that healthy women grow babies too large to birth is a common fallacy in twenty-first-century obstetrics. There is a mistaken belief that small women who mate with big men are especially likely to encounter this problem. In fact, one of the foremost experts on the evolution of the female pelvis, anthropologist Dana Walrath (2003), finds that the mother, not the father, controls the size of her fetus through her DNA. Instead of viewing a woman's pelvis as an impediment to birth, Walrath suggests that we appreciate our birthing apparatus as evolutionarily successful. As the mother of a baby born naturally at 10 pounds, 11 ounces (4.8 kg), I concur. Birthing women are capable of far more than most of us realize.

Explore Your Feelings

Acquiring information about your C-section is not enough. You probably also have many feelings to work through before you will be able to face birth again. Emotional clarity usually requires much soul-searching, tears, feelings of anger and sadness, and a safe outlet for all these. Some women can write in their journals and reach equilibrium. Other women need to talk to a friend or a therapist.

Women's feelings sometimes gather in a storm around the experience of surgery, if it was traumatic, and other times around the events that led to the surgery. Some women feel angry or sad about both. Because these two areas of emotion can be distinct, I explore them separately here.

Emotional Work about the Events Leading to the C-Section

For some women, the surgery itself was not a big deal, but reviewing the events that led to the C-section triggers strong emotions. These women feel that their doctors did not give them full information, that they themselves were too scared about the baby's health to make a rational decision, or that they "wimped out" because the pain was greater than they anticipated.

Of course, the emotions that surround cesarean sections are complicated. Women can feel angry and sad that a surgery happened, and at the same time feel joy and relief that modern medicine saved their lives and the lives of their babies. In the days or weeks after a C-section, well-meaning doctors and friends may have said to "just be happy that your baby is alive and healthy." And in some ways, this focus is appropriate for a new mother as she learns to care for an infant. In preparation for a VBAC, however, the advice is less apt. As a woman prepares to give birth again, she will benefit from acknowledging her feelings about the previous surgery.

About eighteen months after having a C-section, Ellie witnessed the homebirth of her sister's child. Ellie was extremely nervous about attending a homebirth, which she thought of as irresponsible and risky. Yet the experience of watching her sister give birth naturally, with a great deal of support, made her weep for days. "I didn't cry after the C-section. I was much too busy and overwhelmed to even think about whether I was sad. I'd gotten stuck, nothing was happening, they were worried about the baby. It was just a business decision, really. I had no idea how I really felt about it until I saw my sister give birth," she explained tearfully. "Why couldn't I have had that experience?"

The weeping lasted for several days, and after a day or two her husband became worried. He thought she should get professional help. Ellie knew the weeping would end on its own, so she gave herself time and permission to cry. Then she felt better and finally ready to face the idea of another birth.

Now pregnant with her second child, Ellie is planning a VBAC in the hospital. She is still worried that her body "won't be able to do it." But she has a model in her head now of what a natural birth looks like. She thinks she will be much more insistent this time that she get plenty of time to labor. "I just didn't know it could be any other way the first time around," she says.

Writing, talking, and crying are three ways that other women have found release for their feelings about their C-sections. Sometimes, just saying something out loud makes it easier to live with. Whether you talk to a professional counselor, your partner, a doula, or a good friend, making peace with your experience is essential.

Emotional Work about the Surgery

Some women, even those who fully accept their C-sections as medically necessary, feel traumatized by the surgery itself. If this describes your experience, you are far from alone. Medical trauma is the type of overwhelming event that leaves some people with posttraumatic stress disorder (PTSD). It would not be unusual if a traumatic surgical experience brought out some symptoms of PTSD as you head into the next labor (Sperlich & Seng, 2008).

The experience of surgery, not just C-section, causes many people to feel helpless. Your body is literally on display to strangers. A curtain partitions you from your own belly and comes so close to your head that you may feel claustrophobic. "I felt like a trapped animal," remembers one woman.

The attitudes of the doctors and nurses in the operating room may increase your sense of alienation. If the anesthesiologist who stays by your head is silent, you are left to wonder what is happening. Other women report revulsion at listening to doctors converse about irrelevant topics while performing surgery. As a rule, partners are allowed to accompany birthing women to the operating room, but it is usually the partners' first time at a surgery, too. Partners need someone to talk them through the experience as much as birthing mothers do. Although some partners do an excellent job of narrating what they see and helping the birthing woman remain calm, others cannot fill this role.

The physical sensations of surgery are too much for some women to bear. Epidurals are safer for women than general anesthesia, yet being awake during surgery brings with it the fear of being able to feel too much. "I kept telling them I could feel things that I wasn't supposed to feel, but they told me they'd put as much stuff [anesthesia] in me as they could and I couldn't get any more," remembers Sarah. Even if there is no pain, the tugging sensation can make women nauseous. "If you can imagine having surgery on a boat in the middle of a bad storm, that's what it felt like," recalls another woman.

For a variety of reasons, babies born by cesarean often need help to start breathing. Even if you have asked to see your baby immediately after it is born, you may not. "That was the worst part," remembers LaKesha, who gave birth to twins by cesarean. "They took them across the room, I couldn't see either of them, and I didn't know what was happening. No one was talking to me and there wasn't any crying, so I thought they were dead." A few seconds or a few minutes can feel like an eternity when you lie there helplessly wondering what is happening, especially if your partner has left your side to be with the baby. Giving birth by cesarean section can make a woman feel irrelevant to the whole process, a second thought.

You bring all these feelings—of fear, helplessness, irrelevance, loneliness—with you when you leave the operating room. They do not just dissipate in a happy cloud when you reunite with your baby in the recovery room. These feelings can make it extraordinarily difficult to connect with your partner (who not only did not experience the surgery as you did but may have unwittingly helped make it feel degrading to you) and with your baby. You may have extra trouble breastfeeding. You may want to scream at your childbirth-preparation teacher that she did not properly prepare you for birth. Being around other women with new babies, women you assume had different birth experiences, can be excruciating. If you really wanted a natural birth but ended up with a C-section, all these feelings can be compounded by your own judgment that you "failed."

At the next birth, it is vital that you feel supported. The hospital setting itself may cause you much anxiety. For specific ideas and resources to overcome your strong reactions to the hospital, read "Birth for the Survivor of a Traumatic Event," page 115, and also check out some of the books specifically about birth and trauma, such as *Natural Childbirth after Cesarean: A Practical Guide*, by Walters and Crawford, and *Invisible Heroes: Survivors of Trauma and How They Heal*, by Belleruth Naparstek. Naparstek also sells a helpful CD (also available as an MP3 download) called "A Guided Meditation for Healing Trauma (PTSD)." Knowing that you have felt panicked before, you might seek out some new methods of calming yourself, such as meditation or hypnosis.[*]

With the help of someone you trust, make a plan for your VBAC and also for the possibility of a repeat cesarean section. Think through the factors that caused you to feel so overwhelmed or panicked the first time. You might be able to avoid some of them should a second C-section occur. In particular, you might consider seeking special permission to bring a doula or other support person, beyond your partner, with you into the operating room. This person's job would be to help you stay

---

[*] *Hypnosis for birth is not an altered state in which a hypnotist controls your actions. Rather, it is a method of achieving extremely deep relaxation, similar to the way you feel as you are going to sleep or when you are intensely concentrated on an enjoyable task, like putting together a puzzle or reading a novel. Many childbirth education teachers incorporate some instruction on hypnosis and relaxation into their courses. A relaxation CD and a book and website on hypnosis for birth are listed in "Visualization and Meditation Books and CDs," page 267.*

focused and calm. The knowledge that you have planned to change those things that caused you so much pain may produce the serenity you need to relax into giving birth.

Don't Use Pitocin

Some caregivers mistakenly believe that a woman planning a VBAC needs pharmaceutical help to achieve regular, effective contractions. But science has proven that Pitocin and similar drugs are far more dangerous than helpful for VBAC. You will have to be especially adamant about refusing Pitocin if your C-section followed an induction. You—and your caregivers—will need extra patience to make sure you do not repeat that common scenario. If you went a week or more past your due date last time, it will help you, psychologically as well as physiologically, to have a long list of natural induction methods you would be willing to try if your due date approaches and possibly passes. These methods might or might not get labor started, but you will feel as if you are doing something.

Birth for the Survivor of a Traumatic Event

Survivors of traumatic events often find labor and birth especially challenging. Mickey Sperlich, Ph.D., a certified professional midwife, and Julia Seng, Ph.D., a nurse-midwife, research the effects of PTSD on pregnancy, birth, and mothering. Their book, *Survivor Moms* (2008), focuses on women's stories of birthing after sexual abuse; however, their broader research encompasses many kinds of trauma. Traumas that might impinge on your birth experience include abortion, miscarriage, medical trauma, rape, war, interpersonal violence, witnessing violence, being threatened, and experiencing racial discrimination. "For survivors," Sperlich and Seng write, "birth can be a huge challenge because they want it to be a safe and positive experience and a strong start to their mothering. But many aspects of birth itself (e.g., pain, being overwhelmed) and many aspects of birth care (e.g., being touched, losing privacy, not being in control, being overpowered by authority figures) are a reminder or reenactment of abuse" (p. 80).

Natural Ways to Get Labor Started

Eat dates: Studies published in the *Journal of Obstetrics and Gynecology* in 2017 confirm what midwives in some parts of the world have long known: dates have a positive impact on labor. Though the study was relatively small (154 first-time mothers), the effect of dates on labor was so strong that the results were statistically significant even among this small group. This study could not confirm scientifically that labor was brought on faster by eating dates; however, since many of the same hormones and processes are responsible for starting labor as continuing labor, midwives strongly suggest eating dates if you are at all worried about going past your due date.

Brisk walking: Walking can bring on contractions by stimulating your uterus mechanically. If walking by itself does not work, it may work in combination with another natural method.

Nipple stimulation: You can do this yourself, or you can involve your partner. Gently roll, pinch, or pull on both of your nipples at the same time. To bring on labor, you may need to do this for an hour or more continuously.

Acupressure: Professional acupuncturists offer specific treatments to get labor started. You can also browse the Internet for advice about finding your own acupressure points to stimulate labor. YouTube offers several helpful videos, including three by a Brooklyn-based certified doula and licensed acupuncturist, Laurel Axen Carroll. You can find her videos at www.youtube.com/user/Ancientcurrent.

Herbs: Many herbs are known to stimulate labor. Two of the best-known and widely used herbs for this purpose are black cohosh and blue cohosh. These herbs can have a strong effect, so please consult an herbalist or naturopath before taking either of them. They can be purchased at many natural-foods stores or over the Internet. The video *Pregnancy Questions: How to Use Blue and Black Cohosh to Induce Labor*, by Elizabeth Bachner, a licensed midwife and licensed acupuncturist from Los Angeles, is available at: www.youtube.com.

Homeopathic remedies: Many homeopathic remedies can be used to stimulate labor. You can research this through the Internet or in a book about homeopathy or, best of all, you can consult a professional homeopath in your area for personalized recommendations.

Castor oil: Drinking 2 ounces (60 ml) of castor oil makes your intestines cramp. The theory is that these cramps stimulate your uterus and cause it to begin to contract. If the right hormones are present, this will induce labor. Drinking castor oil usually causes diarrhea, however, so this is usually a last-resort remedy. If your water is broken, loose bowel movements could increase your risk of introducing germs into your vagina, so it is not recommended in this case.

Spicy food: Eating spicy food works on the same theory as castor oil. Anything stimulating in the abdominal area might stimulate uterine contractions. This is often dismissed as an "old wives' tale," but I suspect that the "stimulation" effect is real for many women. Many women I interviewed swore this was a key factor in the beginning of their own labors.

Engage in sexual activities and have orgasms: This has also been advised by midwives for a long time, but, perhaps not surprisingly, there are few scientific, rigorous studies about this topic. (Before 2001, there was only one tiny study, with a sample size of just 28 women.) Since then, a few compelling studies have been conducted, and the good news is that sexual activity does appear to shorten the length of pregnancy. We suspect it is either from the uterine activity of tightening during arousal and orgasm or, in the case of heterosexual sex, from effects of semen on a woman's cervix. Both are suspected of playing a role, so one without the other is still worth it. So, unless you are trying to prevent preterm birth, have as much fun as you can, by yourself or with a partner, in the last weeks of pregnancy!

Sperlich and Seng discovered that women with histories of trauma tend to go in one of two directions for birth. Some women are so disturbed at the thought of birth pain, of feeling out of control, or of a baby emerging from the vagina that they would prefer to avoid the birth experience altogether. These women may schedule a C-section or ask for an epidural as soon as they enter the hospital. Other women with a history of trauma desire to feel fully in control of the birth experience. These women are more likely than others to plan a natural birth, even a homebirth, and up to 50 percent more likely to seek midwifery care rather than obstetrical care (Sampselle, 1992). These women are often interested in finding healing of past wounds through giving birth naturally.

Tragically, many survivors experience birth as a new trauma. The pain, the treatment by staff members, or having other people making decisions about their bodies piles new wounds on top of old. The postpartum period with a new infant can be especially difficult after such an experience.

Sperlich and Seng noticed, however, that many other survivors were "deeply healed and strengthened, uplifted and primed to bond with their infants by the experience of being well cared-for or of having simply been . . . triumphant in this challenge" (p. 80). One mother, Shakta, describes her experience this way: "The sensation of giving birth to my daughter was amazing. I use words like 'indescribable,' and I mean it. Physically it felt like rape feels; it hurts so bad that your mind goes away in a shower of sparks. Mentally it was an inversion of that experience. An initiation rather than a violation. When it was all over and the sparks coalesced into thought, I had a baby and the room was awash in sunlight" (p. 110).

If you have experienced past trauma, how do you make sure that you will be among the survivors for whom birth is a healing experience? The difference is in the planning and anticipation. Women who were able to anticipate "what would stir up posttraumatic reactions in them were best able to come through the experience feeling uplifted" (Sperlich & Seng, 2008, p. 80). In your case, bringing a supportive team with you to the hospital is not just a nice idea; it is essential. Many doula training programs give extra attention to special needs like yours. Even if you do not feel comfortable disclosing your history to your caregiver or to a doula, your doula may instinctively understand that you need help to feel in control of your birth experience. A doula can help you achieve as much control and autonomy in labor and delivery as possible, even if this means standing outside your door to protect your right to labor in privacy.

For survivors of sexual abuse, feelings about internal examinations demand special consideration. If you know that internal examinations bring up bad feelings for you, make sure you talk with your care provider about this during pregnancy. Many practitioners do routine vaginal examinations at prenatal visits, especially at a first visit. Some caregivers are more willing than others to forgo internal exams in pregnancy and labor. In labor, they rely on external cues about how labor is progressing. But often internal exams provide important information, and you yourself might want to know how your cervix is doing. So discussing your stress responses ahead of time gives you a chance to come to agreement with your caregivers about techniques or adaptations that would make you feel well cared for, even if you still feel stress.

For all women, birth is a complicated, out-of-the-ordinary event. We all deserve a supportive team and the right to make decisions about our bodies. For some women, because of past experiences or the labeling of their pregnancies as "high-risk," birth is potentially scarier than for others. If you fall into any of these categories of special circumstances—having twins, planning a VBAC, or giving birth after a traumatic event—please make sure you have the support and resources that you need. You and your baby deserve the best possible start together, and there are people out there who feel passionate about helping you achieve it.

Now that you have prepared so well for giving birth naturally, let's explore birth itself.

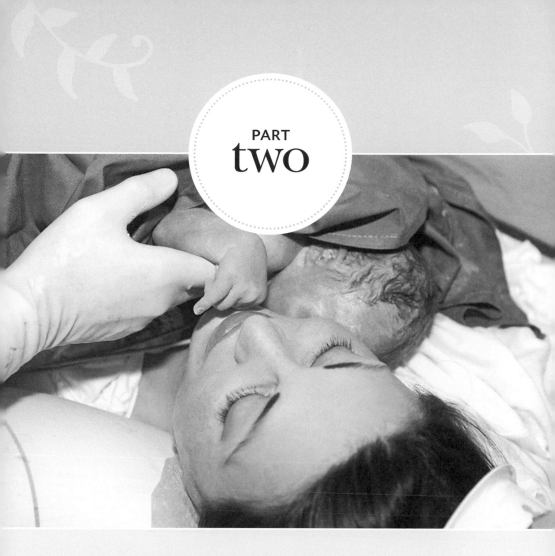

GIVING BIRTH

CHAPTER 6

WHAT LABOR FEELS LIKE: A GUIDE TO SENSATIONS

"**S**O WHAT'S IT REALLY LIKE?" a pregnant woman in her eighth month asked me on the bus in Manhattan. "How bad does it get?" You have probably asked—or wanted to ask—this question of your friends and acquaintances, too. You may have hoped that your childbirth-preparation class would give you a satisfying answer. You notice, somewhat perplexed, that your pregnancy books don't really tell you what to expect.

What is labor like? My short answer, the one I gave to the pregnant woman on the bus, is that my labors were intense. They were painful. And they were the most satisfying things I have ever done. I can honestly say that I enjoy giving birth. Not because I have a high tolerance for pain. I welcome the physical sensations of labor because they make me feel more alive than anything else I have ever experienced. Like a marathon runner, I am proud that I made it to the finish line. That sense of accomplishment and knowledge of what my body can do are worth every minute of pain.

There is certainly far more to say than this about what labor is really like. I am fascinated by women's experiences of labor. In this chapter, I will share with you what I have gleaned as a woman who has given birth, as a doula and childbirth educator in North America, and as an anthropologist in Russia. I will tell you what I have learned by interviewing more than two hundred women about their labors and witnessing another one hundred natural births.

Here's the catch: I can tell you about an average labor. I can tell you what I see most often. Yet, as any rudimentary statistics class shows, the average tells you absolutely nothing about individual cases. More important than the average is the truth that every labor is unique.

How do labors vary? Of course, they vary by time. Some labors are almost too fast to believe; the phases described here last minutes, not hours. Other labors plateau at certain points, so that one phase and set of sensations come to dominate the whole experience.

Labors also vary by intensity. Some women feel no pain. Others feel pain, but it is never stronger than a strong menstrual cramp. Others feel pain so intense that it requires much focused effort to get through. Still others feel pain so excruciating that they are traumatized, even to the point of having fearful flashbacks years later. As the table on page 124 shows, most women fall into the third category, and the next most common category is the second. The experiences of no pain and excruciating pain are extremely rare. I have worked with one woman whose pain seemed extraordinary, and I have interviewed a handful of women who experienced virtually no pain during their labor. The woman who experienced extreme pain had extreme fears and very little preparation. I have met only one woman who experienced a pain-free labor without consciously "doing something" to relieve pain. The others who described little or no pain had all practiced hypnosis for childbirth.

In answering the question "Just how bad does it really get?" I will focus on labor at the third level of intensity—painful contractions that require much focused effort to get through. A full answer to this question can be helpful for fine-tuning your mental and spiritual preparation for natural birth, even if your labor ends up in the second category, of pain like a strong menstrual cramp.

Overpreparation is better than underpreparation. Many natural-birth advocates, including Grantly Dick-Read, Marie Mongan, Sheila Kitzinger, and Ina May Gaskin, believe that eliminating fear can lead to a less painful birth. By preparing yourself well, you may actually have the power to shift yourself from a more painful category to a less painful category.

How Women Describe Labor Pain in Natural Childbirth

Intensity Level	Percentage of Women	Possible Reasons Correlative Factors
No pain	1	Painless natural childbirth occasionally occurs without conscious preparation, but more often these women have used hypnosis, acupuncture, or other special non-drug pain-relieving techniques. They may also be genetically equipped to give birth less painfully than others.
Labor is painful, but never overwhelming. These women may report that childbirth was no more painful for them than other physical experiences, such as strong menstrual cramps, dental work, or a broken bone. They may or may not say they have a high tolerance for pain.	2–7	These women may be genetically equipped to give birth less painfully; they may be less fearful than others about pain, childbirth, or becoming a mother; they may easily slip into a meditative state; or they may have used hypnosis, acupuncture, or other special non-drug pain-relieving techniques. Their babies may be smaller than average and may require less than 10 centimeters of dilation or less effort to push out.
Pain is intense and requires effort (usually, a focus on breathing and relaxing) to get through. Most would agree that labor has been their most painful physical experience. Many compare it with running a marathon.	85–96	Whether labor lasts three or thirty-six hours, this is the way most women who have given birth naturally later describe the pain.
Excruciating, unbearable pain	1–5 (The percentage jumps appreciably if labor is induced.)	Physical or genetic factors may make birth more painful for these women. Excruciating pain is most often associated with a baby who is in an unfavorable position (for instance, the baby's head is tilted or the baby is in the posterior position); a mother with a high level of fear; a mother with an untreated history of sexual, physical, or emotional abuse; or a mother who has experienced other painful trauma.

Finally, labors vary by meaning. What your labor and birth experience means to you will be different from what your neighbor's means to her. Your labor will have different meanings, too, for your midwife or doctor, your mother, and your partner.

Labor Sensations

Though the phases of labor can be so short as to be nonexistent, you will probably feel some or all the sensations described in the following sections building in your body and mind.

Physical Preparation for Labor

Numerous women begin labor days or weeks before giving birth, with a few hours of painless or painful contractions that eventually disappear. The common term for this experience is *false labor* or, more professionally, *Braxton-Hicks contractions* (after the doctor who described them in the nineteenth century). I see this sort of cramping as early, early labor. Your uterus is practicing, just as an athlete practices before a big event. This kind of labor usually happens within three weeks of delivery. Often, these contractions are doing real work, the work of thinning and shortening, or "effacing," the cervix (see the diagram on page 126). When Braxton-Hicks contractions closely match real labor—the contractions are painful and for a while, regular—the uterus will likely be in top shape for the actual event. When I hear a woman describe this sort of experience, I expect that her actual labor is going to go well and relatively fast.

Classically, Braxton-Hicks contractions follow no pattern. You get a contraction, and then three minutes later you have another, and then fifteen minutes later another, and then seven minutes later another, and so on. Usually within about two hours the cramps disappear altogether. Their irregularity tells you that you are probably not yet experiencing progressive labor.

Yet often Braxton-Hicks contractions feel just like the real deal. You may have no way of knowing what's going on until your contractions slow and disappear. This may happen several times over the course of days or weeks, until you are so used to crying wolf that you virtually ignore labor when it finally does arrive. This is frustrating, yet it is nature's excellent method of getting us ready for birth.

Another common experience in prelabor is "bloody show" and the loss of your mucous plug. Your cervix always has an opening in it, but that opening is literally plugged up by thick mucus. This protects your uterus from bacteria. As your cervix begins to open, the tight canal loosens around the mucous plug and it falls out. Also, capillaries near the cervical opening burst and bleed. These events might happen in two stages or in one and in any order. You may see bloody show and then a mucous plug or a mucous plug and then bloody show. First-time mothers are most likely to see bloody show before labor. Women typically notice either of these when they wipe after going to the bathroom. Bloody show is just that: a show of blood. The mucous plug looks like a lot of thick, white mucous that is tinged pink or red.

As a doula, I have been texted many photos of bloody show and mucous plugs from women eager to know whether "this is it." Doulas are used to this; however, I do not recommend posting these photos on social media sites (though I see them there frequently). If it helps you to decide if "this is it," I can tell you that every single photo I have ever been texted has, indeed, been the real deal. So, if you see a show of blood or a mucous-like object in your underwear or on toilet paper, you are noticing a sign of impending labor.

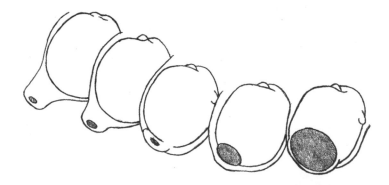

The cervix opens like a turtleneck over the head of the baby. On the far left you can see a uterus at the beginning of labor. The cervix is long and thick. As labor progresses, the cervix gets shorter and thinner and then opens to allow the baby to descend.

Other Prelabor Feelings

Other feelings that you have prior to labor are identifiable only in retrospect. Ah, yes, that irritability I was feeling must have signaled the beginning of labor. Or, my urge to wax all the floors in the house—that was nesting! Women report feeling some, all, or none of the following:

• A nesting instinct

• Irritability

• A strong sense of focus or purpose

• Certainty that "This is the day!"

• A lightening of both body and spirit

• A shedding of fear

• Cramp-like sensations that are annoying, like a low-level headache

Onset of Early Labor

Early-labor sensations are most often described as mild menstrual cramps. Pain is felt low in the abdomen, perhaps centered at the pubic bone. Alternatively, the contraction begins as low back pain and progresses over ten to thirty seconds into menstrual cramp–like abdominal pain. Though this is the most common description of early contractions, some women say that their entire belly feels crampy or that they feel the pain higher in their abdomen. Some women feel only back pain in the beginning.

These early-labor sensations can be accompanied by a rush of fear, excitement, or both. Your body may feel restless. Resting becomes difficult. You are still fully capable of going about daily tasks without much interference.

These feelings may continue at the same pace and intensity for anywhere between five minutes and eight hours. There is no accurate way to predict this time span, especially in a first labor. Your best predictor is your own mother's first labor, though the many factors affecting the length of labor make that a rough guide at best.

Early Labor Builds: 0 to 3 Centimeters

You are now definitely feeling contraction pain in your abdomen, not only in your back. These surges are probably low, near your pubic bone, and they probably build to a peak. As your cervix begins to dilate, the pains are more intense, probably at the level of your average or even strong menstrual cramps. The pain may last as little as ten seconds or as long as a minute. The amount of time between cramps is five to fifteen minutes.

You are probably still capable of walking during a contraction, though perhaps you have to switch to a wider gait. You may want to sway or rock during a contraction, or walk around between contractions and stop to lean on someone or something during contractions. You can still easily move from one place to another (in active labor you will probably get attached to one place and one position and find moving quite difficult).

You are still capable of rational thought. This is a difficult point for many North American women. You are starting to feel more pain and you still have all your wits about you. Your mind can start to spin out if you give it permission. If you are like most women, you will harbor secret or not-so-secret hopes that these sensations signal active labor and that you are already 8 centimeters dilated. You are probably hoping the pain won't get much worse. If you think about this pain continuing for many hours, you can feel hopeless, depressed, and inadequate to the task.

You can counteract such thoughts by staying in the moment. When you wonder about the future of your labor, ask your support team to help you stay in the present. Just deal with the contraction you are in, not the next one or the one after that.

Give your mind something else to focus on besides the pain. If you watch a movie, your brain will be engaged in the story. Every so often a contraction will bring your focus back to your body. You deal with the contraction and then go right back to the movie. If you are making lasagna, again, you focus on cutting, sautéing, and layering. Every so often, you deal with a contraction. Then back to the ricotta cheese. As your contractions progress, you will give them more and more focused attention.

Early Labor: 3 to 5 Centimeters

At some point, you will no longer be able to focus on anything outside of your labor. You turn off the movie, you put away the lasagna ingredients, and you welcome a feeling of fog between contractions. Hormones flooding your system disconnect you from the real world, not just during but even *between* contractions. You start to lose your sense of time. Your detachment deepens with the progress of your labor.

Your contractions feel more intense and more painful than menstrual cramps. Most women find that back pressure or hip squeezing helps tremendously during contractions. Massage and back pressure work best in this stage of early active labor. Counterpressure, on hips or lower back, relieves pain in the same way that squeezing a stubbed toe does.

You will start to get annoyed when your support team asks you questions that require any thought on your part. In active labor you cannot really make choices. Your support team has to switch from asking you whether you would like a drink of water to just offering you a cup with a straw. If you want it, you will sip from it. If you don't want it, you will shake your head no. Instead of saying, "Breathe deeply," your coach might model a long inhalation.

If you can believe that you will feel annoyed when someone asks you whether you want a drink of water, imagine how you will feel if a doctor asks you to make a serious medical decision at this time. Asking a woman in active labor to think rationally about anything interferes with the natural processes at work. It is important to have support people you trust to give your medical caregivers and nurses the answers you would give and ask you only to nod your assent.

Your breathing is likely to change dramatically. During a contraction in this stage of labor, almost every woman naturally alters her breathing, making her breaths longer and deeper.

You will probably notice dramatic differences between contractions that you fight and contractions during which you let go. An instinct to tense up and fight off the pain may arise again and again. If you experiment, you will find that tensing up makes the pain worse. When you consciously relax and surrender to the pain, it is more bearable. You will likely appreciate reminders from your coaches. If your noises become high-pitched and your face or shoulders tense up, your helpers can prompt you to soften your body.

If you are an extrovert, you will probably find some words or phrases coming out of your mouth during your contractions in a repetitive, rhythmic way. I have heard everything from "It hurts, it hurts" to "Ow" to "Oh my God, oh my God, oh my God" to "Help me, please help me." This can be disconcerting to some support people, yet many women seem to benefit from vocalizing this way. Most can easily switch to phrases like "yes, yes, yes" and "now, now, now" or, as in my case, "baby, baby, baby" if their coaches offer these as options. Before labor you might prepare positive, affirming words to use during contractions. It is the making of repetitive sounds that seems important.

Introverts and women who have training in meditation, yoga, hypnotic birth, or other inward-focused arts begin a concentrated journey inward that can be intense to watch from the outside. Support people may feel completely useless because the woman appears to be so far inside herself. This same woman may say later that "I couldn't have done it without you." For such women, having a witness is important in and of itself. Support people "hold the space" and make it "safe" for a woman to lose herself completely.

By the way, until 2014, if your cervical opening measured 4 cm, you were considered in "active labor." But the definition of active labor was changed in 2014 and now hospitals typically only admit women after they have reached 6 cm. This doesn't change how 4 to 5 cm *feels*, though. For many women, 4 to 5 cm really is active labor in the sense that contractions require your full concentration and you loosen your hold on your normal, rational self and begin to feel more floaty and dreamy.

Active Labor: 6 to 7 Centimeters

In this phase, your contractions may or may not feel more intense than they did from 3 to 5 centimeters. They may or may not get longer or closer together. In any case, as you enter active labor you are probably finding your rhythm.

When you have found your rhythm, labor seems to flow smoothly in a predictable pattern. You become so immersed in the ebb and flow of contractions that you lose track of time. Each contraction is intense and demanding, for you and for your support team. Between contractions you probably go deeply inward. You probably keep your eyes closed, and

Natural Ways to Relieve Labor Pain

Massage: This includes feather-light rhythmic touch up and down your back or arms or legs (helpful in all stages of labor); massaging your hands, feet, shoulders, or lower back (usually in early to early active labor); rubbing your temples; and massaging your head.

Hip squeezing: Standing behind you, someone squeezes the tops of your hips inward during contractions.

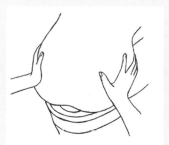

You can use the hip squeeze to help handle labor pain while standing, sitting on an exercise ball, sitting at the edge of your bed, or sitting backward on the toilet, as shown. These positions allow your partner the best access to your back.

Back pressure: Using fists or one or two tennis balls, your support person pushes into your lower back during contractions. This is especially useful when the back of the baby's head is pressing against your spine (this "posterior position" occurs in a small percentage of labors).

Change of position: While the act of changing position may increase your pain, the new position itself may relieve pain. Good positions to try include all-fours (especially for relieving back pain and encouraging a baby to change position), sitting on a birthing ball, leaning forward on a chair with a backrest, and leaning against another person, the wall, or a piece of furniture.

Walking: Pacing a room or taking a walk helps many women.

Water: For many women, water is the best pain reliever. You can stand in the shower so the water streams on your back or your abdomen. If that is too intense, you may be able to position a chair so that only your legs and feet are showered. Or you can soak in warm water in a tub.

(continued)

Heat and cold: Use cold, damp cloths on your face (this is especially helpful during transition). Use heat, or alternate heat and cold, on the lower back. The heat and cold can come from commercial products for one-time use, heating pads, ice packs, chilled cans of soda, or damp cloths that are microwaved or left in the freezer for a while.

Words of encouragement: Certain words or phrases can work wonders. Your birth team can try these:

- I love you.
- You're safe.
- You're amazing.
- You're really doing it.

- You're having a baby!
- You're my hero.
- You're such a great mom.
- I'm so proud of you.

Visualization: If you have planned this ahead of time, your birth team can whisper a word or phrase to remind you to use visualization during a contraction. Some common visualizations involve opening flowers, waves, beaches, and forests. If you have not planned a visualization, your birth team can talk you through one. (See page 181 for examples of visualization scripts.)

Breathing: Concentrate on breathing deeply and evenly.

Crying: Crying can help you "let go" during labor. Women whose contractions prior to a crying episode are quite painful often find them less so after the release of tears.

you may even doze off between contractions. You do not interact much with the outside world. By this time, all the team members know their parts. When you say, "It's starting," you and everyone else in the room assume your roles and positions, like actors on a stage.

A nurse or doctor who comes in during this phase seems like an intruder in a private world. Everyone inside the world notices how uninitiated the outsider seems. The outsider's voice is likely to seem especially loud.

Doing anything beyond handling contractions seems like a huge ordeal. Moving into a new position feels daunting. Drinking a sip of water feels like a heroic task. Getting to the bathroom to pee deserves an Olympic gold medal.

When the nurse puts a Doppler on your belly to measure the baby's heartbeat, you probably hardly notice. Likewise, when she sticks a thermometer into your mouth. As long as you, yourself, don't have to do anything, events don't register much on your radar screen.

The difference in painfulness between contractions you fight and contractions to which you surrender is even larger than it was earlier. Any anxiety or fear that causes you to tense can make contractions feel unbearable.

If you are committed to a natural birth and you have had any training in deep relaxation (such as yoga, meditation, or hypnosis), you are likely to respond very well to simple commands and statements from your support team: "Just focus on this contraction," "Just get through this one," "You can do it," "I love you," "Squeeze my hand to get through this," "Go low," "Ride through this wave." Your brain has only a tiny thread of a connection to the outside world. If the connection is full of fear, your pain will get out of control. If your connection to the real world is full of calm reassurance, you can go about your task of letting go.

Transition: 8 to 10 Centimeters

For some women, transition is no more intense than labor from 3 to 5 centimeters' dilation or 5 to 7 centimeters' dilation. For most, though, transition is more intense than all that has preceded it. For those who experience a shift in intensity, this part of labor demands complete surrender. During transition, the rational mind is wholly subsumed. It feels disconnected from the body. Some women describe transition as an out-of-body experience, in which they feel themselves floating above their bodies, watching what is happening.

You are likely to keep your eyes closed all the time. If you are in water or have found a very comfortable position, you might relax very deeply or even doze between contractions.

Very little information from the material world can break through to your brain. Your support team may be conversing in the corner, but you are completely oblivious. Your husband may leave for a moment to scarf down a bagel, and you hardly notice that the nurse or doula has taken his place. Later, you will swear he never left your side. Your medical care-givers may suggest interventions that you would or would not welcome, yet you can scarcely pay them any attention. Decision making feels dreamlike, not businesslike.

Women make dramatic statements during transition. Among the more common ones are "I feel like I'm breaking in two" and "I feel like I'm dying." Sometimes, a woman will cry, "I'll never be the same!" Such statements can have a profound impact on partners and other support people who are not prepared for them. If they are prepared, they can recognize these words as a sign of transition. They can begin their own internal shift from supportive waiting to active anticipation of pushing and birth.

Dramatic statements reflect the profound shift that is happening internally. When I talk to women after labor, most tell me that at the moment these words escaped their lips, they were already accepting the sensations. In other words, when a woman says, "I feel like I'm dying," she is probably just surrendering to labor, not pleading for help. Her rational mind, full of fear of death, has tried to reengage at this point. Yet, for most of us, rationality is long gone. We face death (or, in this case, the idea of death) more sanguinely without logic.

At this point in my labors, I lost any memory of life outside of "Labor Land." Any thoughts that I could not continue were powerless before the inexorable pull of bodily sensations that just kept going, no matter what I thought. Life was not a concept that had any relevance; neither was death. They were thoughts and words, but they did not have the power of physical sensation.

Yes, transition can be difficult, painful, and, for some, soul-wrenching. Yet it means that you are on the cusp of giving birth. When you surren-der to the thought that you might die or break open, that your body is being wrecked, you do come out on the other side. Into . . .

Pushing

For most women, pushing is a relief. During early and active labor your main job was to relax and allow your contractions to open your cervix. When your cervix is fully open, you finally get to use muscles that you can control. About half of your mind returns from the sleepy, dreamy, otherworldly place it has been. A small yet significant percentage of women find pushing to be even harder than cervical dilation. These women say they expected relief at this stage and felt unprepared for the intensity of pushing.

The sensation of pushing is exactly what the word describes. You have an overwhelming urge to bear down. To grunt. The vast majority of women experience this as similar to the feeling of having to expel a large bowel movement.

The sensation is intense, and pushing can be painful. However, because it is more purposeful and conscious than dilation, it can feel more rewarding. You may be able to feel the progress of your baby down the birth canal. My babies' heads felt hard and round as they moved earthward, much more like a duckpin bowling ball than a bowel movement.

Countless women find pushing on a toilet helpful, despite what some nurses say. I've heard it often: "You don't want to give birth on a toilet, do you?" To which the answer is "No, I just want to push here for a while!" As Patty Brennan, a midwife and doula trainer, reminds aspiring doulas, "We are physiologically conditioned to release those muscles when we sit on a toilet." Since many women poop at least once while they are pushing, sitting on the toilet is convenient.

I have heard people say that pushing out a baby is like pushing a grand piano across a room: just that hard and just that satisfying. It can feel wonderful to put your whole body into the effort and to feel the piano start to move, to inch along the floor, to gather momentum. This is very much what the pushing phase of labor feels like.

You are likely to find a position that feels comfortable for you that you will want to use throughout this phase. It may or may not be the position you imagined yourself assuming. Especially if you are squatting or sitting, you will probably want to pull on something as a counterbalance to your pushing. That something may be your support person's shoulders, a rope or bar hanging from the ceiling, or a piece of heavy furniture.

Psychologically, this stage usually feels quite different from all the labor before it. As your cervix opened, you likely dropped further and further into an altered state of consciousness (that floaty feeling of "Labor Land"). Now, as your uterus changes function (instead of pulling open, the top of your uterus now pushes downward), you return to a more rational, awake state. When I am a doula, I often notice that women are more able to converse and participate in banter with staff than they were before.

Your sense of time is still severely distorted during this phase. Though some women push until they are truly exhausted, many women find that the pushing phase goes by too fast. They feel unprepared for the sudden transition from labor to a baby in their arms. Support people can help by reminding you that your baby is almost here, that you are (probably) minutes away from holding your baby. A support person can help direct your attention away from your physical sensations (as overwhelming as they may be) toward your psychological preparation for the big moment.

Birth

Now, your doctor or midwife can see the baby's head. First, it is a sliver that seems to take one step forward, two steps back. Gradually, though faster than you can believe, it emerges fully. All your fears of tearing may come to you in a flood. Or, more likely, you will forget any such fear in your desperate desire to have the baby *out* of your body.

Your vaginal tissues stretch to emit your baby's head. The slower your baby descends, the more time your tissues have to adjust and stretch. That's why, at the very end, your caregiver is likely to say, "Stop pushing!" several times and ask you to blow or pant through contractions. Just an extra second or two can sometimes make a big difference in allowing your tissues to stretch rather than tear. This is not easy! Everything in you is saying, "Push! Push!"

Our vaginas are made with folds and folds of tissue inside. These folds allow the vagina to expand to fit a baby's head. Although the stretching sensation is intense, it is not the same as if your anus or other bodily tissue were being asked to stretch as much. The vagina's accordion-like design allows it to bounce back into shape within hours or days of giving birth.

Many women expel small amounts of poop when they push. This is often something pregnant women desperately fear; in reality, they are usually completely unaware of it happening in the moment. Nurses and caregivers just fold the blue pads over or put a new one down. Voila! The problem is solved in one second and most mothers and partners never even know.

As the baby emerges from your vagina, the sensation is usually one of burning. It is often referred to as the Ring of Fire. If you hook your fingers in the sides of your mouth and stretch your lips, you will know what it is like. Some women are more terrified of this moment than of any other part of labor. They are often unaware of how fleeting the moment really is. Count "one one-thousand, two one-thousand, three one-thousand," and you will know how quickly the burning may pass. For most women, the Ring of Fire lasts three to fifteen seconds. In a rare case, it might last as long as thirty seconds, as you wait for the next contraction to build. Coming after hours of contractions and pushing and just a moment before the Big Moment of birth, this sensation of burning is usually nothing more than a footnote to the experience of labor.

Once your baby's head is out, you may need to give one to three more pushes to get out the body. Or it may come sliding right out. If the baby's shoulders get stuck, your caregiver may ask you to change position quickly and push. When the shoulders pass through the vaginal opening, there may be another tiny twinge of burning. But as the body is born you will probably experience a warm, slippery feeling of intense relief.

And amazing joy. Your baby is born! Yet still attached to you. Which is a pretty good metaphor for the rest of your life.

CHAPTER 7

EARLY LABOR: AT HOME

THE PREVIOUS CHAPTER SHOWED YOU all labor and birth in a snapshot. This chapter and the rest of Part Two will give you a more detailed, stage-by-stage guide to labor. My goal is to help you develop concrete strategies to maintain your guiding principles as you experience labor, from early labor at home through birth in a hospital.

Your commitment to birthing naturally will likely come up against cultural, institutional, interpersonal, and personal obstacles. How will you handle these challenges? These chapters will discuss common barriers in the nitty-gritty detail that you and your support team need. But it's not enough to read about these topics. I encourage you to use the information here to draw up your own questions for your childbirth-preparation classes and for your caregiver. If you are like most women, you will need to talk about these topics in a good amount of detail before you'll feel peaceful, satisfied, and fully prepared for labor.

Ignore Early Labor

Whether your early labor is short or long, my advice to you is to *ignore early labor!*

Labor is usually a long process. Early labor could last one hour, or it could last twenty-four hours or longer. Most first-time moms can't wait for birth to begin, so they get overly enthusiastic about early contractions—the beginning of a long-awaited labor! As cramping pain becomes regular, they often start using pain-management techniques such as conscious breathing.

However, the best pain-management technique you can use in early labor is pretending you're not in labor. Although it makes sense to alert your partner and possibly your caregiver, you will do best to save all your attention for active labor. How will you know when you've reached this stage? It will be when you can no longer talk to anyone except in monosyllables between contractions. In my experience, this sign has been unmistakable. Whether labor is fast or slow, when a woman has trouble concentrating on a conversation between contractions, she has moved beyond early labor. This chapter is about what to do before you get to that point.

Is It Labor?

How will you know that you are in early labor? The short answer is you won't, until afterward. In a short labor, you will know you are in labor because the active part comes on quickly. In an average or longer labor, you will know you are in labor because the low-level signs continue for several hours.

Early labor is often described as uterine contractions that

- are strong enough to feel uncomfortable (they might feel like light to heavy menstrual cramps, and they might involve some back pain);

- occur at definite intervals, usually between three and ten minutes apart (if your contractions are fifteen minutes apart, this may also be early labor, but it is probably *very* early labor); and

- have been regularly spaced or getting closer together for two hours.

Though early contractions might be quite painful, the pain usually lets up completely between contractions. In early labor, you will probably be able to maintain a conversation with another person. Almost certainly you

A Special Case

If your waters break but you are not feeling any contractions, you **are** in labor. Subtle contractions broke your bag of waters; you just aren't feeling them yet. However, you are in a special category of laboring women now: in labor but waiting for contractions. This is a perfectly normal and wonderful way to begin labor. See Chapter Eight for more details.

will be able to talk between contractions. You may even be able to talk during a contraction. If you can talk or walk during a contraction, I encourage you to do so. Your body will demand your attention when it is needed.

When labor comes on fast and furious, a woman's body may commandeer her complete attention to labor almost from the get-go. This is far more common in second and subsequent pregnancies. If it happens to you, most of the advice in this chapter will not apply to you. You have graduated to the next chapters, on active labor!

In first pregnancies, though, labor usually comes on slowly and gradually. In a slower labor, a woman's body gives her time to adjust, mentally and physically. Giving all her attention to her bodily sensations when her body is not yet demanding it has a profound and generally negative effect on a woman's experiences of labor. It makes labor seem long, to the woman and to everyone around her. She may use up her inner resources too early and feel fatigued and drained when it's time to push. And her support team, having rushed in to offer support too early, is also exhausted and drained for the most demanding parts of labor. Because everyone has been looking at the clock for too many hours, there is more likely to be a sense that "this is taking too long; maybe we should do something."

This simple problem is easily avoided. Ignore early labor!

I do not mean that you should entirely block out the fact that you are in labor. I mean that you should purposely give your attention to something else.

As soon as you start to feel contractions, I suggest that you drink a full glass of water. Dehydration can cause your uterus to cramp. If that is what is happening, and labor isn't actually beginning, drinking a glass of water can reveal the truth. If labor is truly beginning, it's a good idea to start well hydrated anyway.

Before labor, in late pregnancy, I encourage you to make a list (with your partner, if you have one) of twenty things you could do in early labor—ten for a daytime labor, and ten for a nighttime labor. These are your last moments of cognizant alone or together time without a baby! From the time you go into active labor until your baby is born, you probably will not remember many details. So your memories of your baby's birthday will mostly come from this early-labor period. Why not plan to do something special and meaningful at this time? It will become a wonderful part of your child's birth story: "On the day you were born, Mommy and Daddy woke up and made cupcakes. We put candles in them and wrapped them up and then we ate them with Grandma and Grandpa after you were born, when you were two hours old."

Daytime Labor

Your daytime list could include activities such as

- going for a walk;
- watching a movie (I know one couple who watched their wedding video and ate popcorn);
- having a candlelight lunch together, at home or at a restaurant;
- playing a board game;
- making a birthday cake;
- making a meal for later (you can freeze it for when you come home from the hospital or bring it with you to eat right after the baby is born);
- putting photos in a photo album (you might save some or all your pregnancy photos for this occasion); and
- meditating. (Even if you do not meditate regularly, you could plan to do a full-body relaxation-visualization that your partner reads out loud to you, perhaps using Maureen Garth's *Starbright* or

Earthlight, books designed for children that contain visualizations perfect for beginners of all ages.)

Walking is my first suggestion because it combines the benefits of conversation or meditative silence with labor enhancement. Walking is a time-honored method of augmenting and maintaining labor.

Eating in early labor is also a good idea. This is your chance to nourish your body for the marathon ahead. Think like a runner: Give your muscles carbohydrates and protein for the job they are about to do. Once you switch into active labor, you will probably have no appetite, so now may be your only chance. If labor is coming on rapidly, you may have no appetite from an early point. In this case, I recommend honey-sweetened, warm (but not hot) herbal tea to give you a few calories and hydration.

Nighttime Labor

If labor starts at night, give yourself about half an hour to gauge what kind of labor you are in.

Scenario 1: Light, Early Labor at Night

If your contractions are mild or spaced more than ten minutes apart, or both, my advice is to *stay in bed and rest* as long as possible. You can give a heads-up phone call to anyone who will be attending your baby's birth: friends, family, midwife, or doula. Don't be enticed to spend much time on the phone, though. Have a glass of water and get back to bed. This rest will give you strength later, when labor gets active.

This goes for your partner, too, no matter how excited the two of you are. By far, the best thing you can do for yourselves is to rest, even if this means lying in bed awake with your eyes closed.

If the contractions are strong enough to keep you from dozing off, or if they keep waking you up, you might take a warm bath to try to calm them down. Many midwives with whom I have worked advocate drinking a glass of wine in this situation. One midwife explains that a glass of wine tends to "knock out early labor" and help a woman get to sleep. In her experience, women who try this remedy get a night of sleep and wake up in the morning in or near active labor. If after nine months of abstinence you don't feel comfortable with this recommendation, a mug of chamomile tea or hot milk might be a good substitute for the wine.

Scenario 2: More Intense Early Labor at Night

If your contractions are relatively strong or close together, I still suggest giving sleep a try. If it is at all possible, rest is your best option. Rest. Rest some more.

Sometimes, however, sleep is impossible. You are in labor, and you cannot rest. Your list of activities for nighttime can include any or all those suggested for the daytime. Taking a walk is just as good for promoting nighttime labor as it is for daytime labor, so if you live somewhere where you can walk outside at night, go ahead. Or stick with relaxing, restful activities, such as

- a warm bath or shower;

- a back massage with oil (for relaxation, not pain management);

- a massage of your feet, hands, legs, arms, and face;

- watching a movie in bed;

- having your partner read a book out loud to you; and

- writing your baby a letter, just to say happy birthday or to describe your goals and values as a parent.

Sex in Early Labor

In midwifery there is a famous saying: "The same energy that got the baby in will get the baby out." Some women find the sensuality of labor, especially of early labor and the pushing stages, to also be quite sexual. As Peggy O'Mara (2003, p. 158) reminds us, "There are many parallels between lovemaking and birth. The senses become acute in both experiences. . . . The same hormone, oxytocin, is released during both lovemaking and labor." If kissing or other lovemaking appeals to you in early labor, go for it! Nipple stimulation is used all over the world as a way to induce or augment labor.

If your bag of waters has broken, however, you should probably exclude any form of vaginal penetration. Without the protection of the amniotic sac, your baby and uterus are vulnerable to infections that can be introduced through the vagina.

When Should You Go to the Hospital?

This is the million-dollar question! First-time mothers sometimes ask it with what seems like desperation. They want a concrete, easy-to-understand, definitive answer, and that is what most hospitals and doctors try to give. The answer usually sounds like this: "When your contractions have been regular and five minutes apart for at least an hour."

This rule of thumb assumes a number of things, however. It assumes that you are the average hospital client, who wants an epidural as soon as possible. It assumes that you have no one with experience who can gauge your labor outside of the hospital. I suggest instead that you go to the hospital when it is the right time for you, not when your labor meets certain criteria.

Go to the hospital whenever you are certain that you should, for physical or emotional reasons or both. An inner voice may tell you adamantly in early labor that you will be safer in the hospital. Once I worked with a first-time, single mother who was 100-percent committed to natural birth. She was at home with unsupportive family members when her waters broke. I tried to convince her to stay at home until strong and regular contractions kicked in. After half an hour on the phone, I understood that the lack of support she felt at home was worse for her than the possibility of interventions in the hospital. She was more willing to contest the hospital staff (who told her right away that she didn't "need to be in all this pain") than her own family. Going to the hospital in early labor was right for her. Please be willing to listen to yourself above all else.

Since you are reading this book, you are working hard to attain a natural birth. You have probably heard or read that staying home as long as possible during labor increases your chances of avoiding interventions and of having a natural birth. This is true. You have chosen to give birth in a hospital, though, so you probably are anxious not to wait too long and risk an unintended homebirth.

You are looking for the magic recipe that will allow you to stay home for most of early and active labor yet arrive at the hospital before you feel the urge to push. Ideally, you will arrive at the hospital when you are about 7 centimeters dilated.

When you arrive at the right time, your labor will be fully established and won't be negatively impacted by arriving at the hospital. The distraction of a new place and new people won't slow down your body's work. Also, you will already know which techniques help you handle contractions and which do not. You will not need to figure this out in the hospital. When Bridget, the woman whose story is told on pages 146 to 147, went into labor, she gave herself many hours to find her labor rhythm at home before she went to the hospital. Her coping techniques were so well established that the hospital personnel checked her vital signs and otherwise left her alone. When a woman is "in the zone," nurses tend to do this. When a woman arrives who is having difficulty handling contractions, nurses are more likely to stay in the room and offer suggestions, even if a support team is present. Nurses and everyone else in a labor room can instinctively tell the difference between a woman who is experiencing pain but who has found her groove and a woman who is experiencing pain and can't get a handle on it.

Strategy Number 1: Get Help with This Decision

It is very hard to gauge your own labor if you haven't had a baby before. Without help, you are not likely to be able to tell how far dilated you are and how much longer labor is likely to be. Your best bet is to have a midwife or doula come to your home to assess your labor. Midwives and doulas have different sets of skills, but either can help determine when it is time to go to the hospital. If you have made no arrangements with a midwife or doula, try to find a friend who has given birth naturally to help. If you would prefer to rely on your partner to fulfill this role, please assure yourself that your partner has read and understood this chapter and has taken notes in your childbirth-preparation classes.

A midwife or doula will probably ask you to talk on the phone through a contraction before she drives to your home. Listening to how you breathe and talk during and between contractions provides a gold mine of information. If you can still talk during a contraction, your midwife or

Facing Pressure to Induce Labor: Bridget's Story

When a woman passes her due date without starting labor, her caregivers may worry that her placenta will stop functioning optimally and that the baby will not receive all the nutrients and oxygen that he needs. Her caregivers may also worry about the baby's size. In Bridget's case, an ultrasound near the end of pregnancy indicated that she might be carrying a large baby. Because a bigger baby requires more opening of the cervix and more pushing, Bridget's nurse-midwives urged her to schedule an induction near her due date.

At the end of pregnancy, most women are psychologically ready to be done with the waiting. When caregivers warn that "this baby may be getting too big to come out of your pelvis" or "the placenta starts to break down when you go past your due date," many women find it hard to insist on waiting for nature to take its course. Bridget's midwives were likely trying to make sure that Bridget and her husband, Eric, had all the facts. They no doubt supported her desire for a natural birth. By expressing their concerns about the size of the baby, suggesting an induction, and even raising the specter of a C-section, they were conscientiously doing their jobs. Bridget, however, experienced their words as "fear and pressure."

Luckily, Bridget and Eric were willing to do significant research into the issues at hand. They also activated their support network. They consulted with their doula, their childbirth-preparation teacher, and Bridget's mother. These people helped them sort through their feelings and the facts. Bridget decided she could wait for nature to take its course. She tried to help nature along with noninvasive techniques such as long walks, acupuncture, and spicy Thai and Italian food.

Bridget's due date came and went with no signs of labor. Her midwives scheduled "nonstress tests" (NST) of the baby every few days. (A nonstress test involves monitoring the baby's heartbeat, at rest and when the baby moves, to make sure the baby is healthy.) At the midwives' insistence, Bridget scheduled an induction with Pitocin for fourteen days past her due date. Ten days past her due date, Bridget allowed one of the midwives to "strip" her membranes, a common procedure in which a practitioner rubs a finger just inside a woman's cervix. This procedure can be mildly or moderately uncomfortable, but it is one of the least invasive of the medical induction methods. Bridget also had a final acupuncture treatment on this day.

Around 12:30 the next afternoon, Bridget started to feel inconsistent contractions. By 2 p.m., the contractions were strong and only three minutes apart. She labored at home for ten hours with the help of Eric, her mother, and their doula before going to the hospital.

In triage, they found out that she was 4 centimeters dilated. She labored for about six more hours in the hospital, in and out of a whirlpool tub and shower. The hospital staff left them alone except for monitoring the baby's heart rate and Bridget's blood pressure. The nurses understood that Bridget was committed to giving birth naturally, and they could see that Eric, Bridget's mother, and the doula were providing all the necessary labor support.

When Bridget felt like pushing, Eric helped her with a squatting position, by sitting behind her and supporting her under her arms. As the baby came down the birth canal, the doula and midwives held warm compresses against Bridget's perineum. It turned out that the baby was on the large side, at 9 pounds, 11 ounces (4.4 kg), but Bridget was quite capable of birthing her naturally. "It was beautiful when she was born!" remembers Bridget. "They put her on my chest, and she nursed immediately, and Eric was sitting behind me and cut her umbilical cord. It was amazing!"

Without substantial information gathering and the support of her team, there is a good chance that Bridget, like nearly 40 percent of women in the United States, would have had her labor induced with pharmaceutical drugs. Instead, with confidence in her body's ability to do what it needed to do, and with the support of Eric, her doula, her mother, and her childbirth-preparation teacher, Bridget was able to face the last days of a longer-than-average pregnancy with equanimity. Bridget did not insist on a natural start to pregnancy no matter what. But she did insist that she would require a real, not a potential, reason to induce labor. Her story illustrates how much support following the natural route can require.

doula is likely to say, "It sounds like you are in early labor. Try this, this, and this. Then let's talk again in a few hours or sooner if your contractions change dramatically in intensity." If your contractions are strong enough to demand your full attention and alter your breathing, your midwife or doula will probably want to see you right away. If your waters have broken, other considerations may or may not come into play at this time.

If you have a midwife. A midwife can help you gauge where you are in labor by performing a vaginal exam. In some areas, hospital midwives are willing to make home visits. Fewer midwives are willing to do this now, however, than in past decades. The next-best choice is to meet the midwife at her office, not at the hospital, if you are having trouble deciding how far along you are.

If you have a doula. A doula who has attended *at least* twenty-five births (preferably more) will be able to give you an educated guess about where you are in labor and when it is time to go to the hospital. A doula will rely on external signs, not a vaginal exam.

If you have a good friend. A good friend who has given birth naturally will probably be able to help you gauge your labor. She will likely remember the difference between early and active labor and be able to help you figure out where you are and when it is time to go to the hospital. A woman who has given birth only with an epidural, though, will not have the "body memory" to help you.

Strategy Number 2: Figure Out Your Labor Patterns

If you don't have a midwife, doula, or experienced friend who can assess your labor in your home, it is up to you and your partner to do this. Here are questions to ask yourself:

• How long have you been feeling contractions?

• How far apart were they when you began to feel them?

• How long did the contractions last when you began to feel them?

• How far apart are the contractions now?

• How long do they last now?

- How fast or how slowly have the contractions you feel increased in intensity or regularity?

(Note: The time between contractions is measured from the onset of one contraction to the onset of the next.)

The answers to these questions will help you understand your personal labor pattern. If you can gauge whether your labor is proceeding quickly or slowly, you will have a better idea about when to go to the hospital. Generally speaking, the way that your labor begins gives some clues about how the rest of labor is likely to proceed. In other words, if early labor is relatively slow and gradual, active labor is also likely to be slow and gradual. If early labor is swift, active labor is likely to follow suit. Of course, there are labors that defy this rule. Remain alert for the signs of active labor (how you act between contractions), and you will catch the drift of your unique labor.

Following are three examples. The goal in all the following scenarios is to arrive at the hospital after your cervix has dilated to at least 6 centimeters.

Scenario 1

If contractions begin lightly, spaced fifteen to thirty minutes apart, and if over a period of five or more hours they gradually become more intense and closer together, until they are five minutes apart, your labor is following a fairly average pattern. You can *probably* count on another six to twelve hours of labor. In other words, you probably should not be in any rush to get to the hospital.

As labor progresses, a good gauge for your partner is your behavior between contractions. At around 4 to 5 centimeters of dilation, you will probably start focusing fully on your labor, and you will lose the ability to joke or hold a conversation between contractions. From this point forward, on average, a woman's cervix dilates 1 to 1½ centimeters per hour, though the normal variation is huge. Once you start focusing fully on your labor, you might give yourself two hours more of laboring at home and then head to the hospital.

Another gauge of where you are in labor is your ability to walk. Women can usually walk between contractions longer than they can talk. If you have been walking between contractions, you may suddenly stop at about 6 to 7 centimeters. At this time, you will be so fully focused on labor that you become rooted to one spot, unwilling to move. When this happens, it is probably time to consider going to the hospital.

I hope you are getting the message that a woman's behavior between contractions is often more indicative of her progress than her behavior during a contraction.

Scenario 2

If contractions come on suddenly and intensely *and* if they occur close together (every five minutes or less) *and* if they increase in intensity, duration, and frequency over the course of the first hour or two or three, you are probably looking at a shorter labor than most. In this case, you should consider giving yourself about one hour from the onset of active labor before you go to the hospital.

Scenario 3

If contractions come on lightly and take many hours to increase in intensity, *or* if contractions are persistent but irregularly spaced (sometimes they are five minutes apart, sometimes they are fifteen minutes apart, sometimes seven minutes, and so on), *or* if they are regular but spaced more than seven minutes apart, your body is probably going about birth at a leisurely pace. In your case, even more than for women with fast labors, staying at home and allowing active labor to establish itself at its own pace is very important if you want a natural birth.

Follow your early-labor plans for daytime or nighttime labor (see pages 141 to 143) for the first three to five hours that you are feeling contractions. If after this time contractions have not increased greatly in intensity or regularity, switch gears.

Whether your labor is beginning during the day or during the night, a longer labor requires more stamina. You need as much rest as possible between contractions. Though there is no scientific way to measure the amount of pain a woman endures during labor, anecdotal evidence suggests that a longer labor is not necessarily more painful but is more exhausting. The challenge for you will be physical and emotional fatigue.

When you haven't produced a baby after what seems like an eternity of contractions, you may understandably feel discouraged. When you have been awake continuously for more than seventeen hours, you will be tired. The longer you are awake, the more tired you will become.

Your task in labor is to rest, rest, and rest! If early labor is giving you time between contractions, try to doze off. If you do not need to use pain-management techniques to get through a contraction, stay in bed with your pajamas on. Review the section on nighttime labor (page 142) for other suggestions.

Your goal is to establish active labor at home before you get to the hospital. In your case, this means that active labor—the kind of labor that takes your breath away and keeps you focused between contractions—goes on for at least three hours. Contractions may still be widely spaced, but if the interval between them remains constant or narrows over three to four hours of more intense labor, you are well on your way. Once active labor has been established over the course of several hours, you can have more confidence that the transition to the hospital won't knock out your labor.

How Long Will Labor Last?

How long does labor last for most women? As you have no doubt garnered from stories of family and friends, the normal range is wide. A 2-hour labor is normal and so is a 28-hour labor. A study by Sandra K. Cesario (2004) found normal labor (with no pharmaceutical augmentation) to range from 1.9 to 34 hours.

Until they experience labor themselves, most women are not aware of the very big and important difference between early and active labor. The super-long labors you have heard about (of your friend who labored for two days, or that woman at work who had a thirty-hour labor) probably involved an active stage of less than eleven hours. Usually, very long labors involve many hours of early labor (up to twenty-three, according to recent studies). This means that contractions are light and far apart for most of the labor. This doesn't mean long labors are easy to deal with. But it means that women do not experience the intensity of active labor as long as we might fear when we hear these horror stories.

Types of Labor, Categorized by Length

Precipitous birth: This is a super-fast, hold-on-for-the-ride labor that lasts under three hours from start to finish. If you are having such a labor, you probably will not have time to consult this book at any point. You may or may not make it to the hospital on time. The good news is that in such situations everything is working so well that an out-of-hospital birth, even unplanned, usually turns out very well.

Average: Most labors, as you might expect, fall into this middle category. In an average labor, you can expect early and active labor to add up to eleven to sixteen hours.

Longer: Some women go about labor at a leisurely pace. For them, early labor can last up to twenty hours and active labor up to twelve.

What Is Happening in Your Body?

If you look at the illustration on page 126, you will see that four-fifths of the dilation phase (early plus active labor) is getting to *3 centimeters'* dilation. Your cervix starts out looking like a turtleneck, with the neck hanging down. The first step of labor is effacement, the shortening and thinning of the cervix. When the cervix is effaced, the turtleneck is no longer hanging down but is pulled tightly against the baby's head. Effacement may happen over a period of days or weeks with no noticeable symptoms. When you begin to feel labor contractions, your cervix may already be partially or fully effaced. Or your cervix may begin to efface only when you begin to feel contractions. In the latter case, your labor may (or may not!) turn out to be a bit on the long side. For this reason, if you have experienced a long early labor and arrive at the hospital to find that you are "only" 3 centimeters dilated, take heart!

Early labor consists of effacement plus the first 3 centimeters of cervical opening. This part of labor takes the longest, yet it also takes the least effort. Active labor is much shorter, yet it takes a great deal more effort.

CHAPTER 8

A VARIATION ON EARLY LABOR:
WHEN YOUR WATERS BREAK BEFORE CONTRACTIONS

Welcome to the "water breaking to start labor" club! You are among an elite membership. Contrary to what Hollywood would have us believe, only one in about ten full-term labors begins with a splash or a leak (Hiersch et al., 2017). Membership in this club has its benefits and drawbacks. The clearest benefit is that you can be certain (unlike the woman trying to figure out whether she is in labor or just experiencing Braxton-Hicks) that you will have your baby in your arms in short order, usually within forty-two hours. You are on your way.

The medical term for your situation is *prelabor rupture of the membranes* or *PROM*. Actually, the breaking of your waters means you *are* in labor, though you do not feel contractions yet. Uterine movements broke your bag of waters, and it is only a matter of time before you will feel them. A sense of confidence that you are, in fact, in labor can be very important. When hospital personnel tell you that you have to "get into labor" within a certain period of time, remind yourself that their terminology is off. You *are* in labor; you just don't feel it yet.

In many cases, when a woman's bag of waters breaks she starts to feel contractions immediately or within a few hours. If this happens to you, and then your labor proceeds in a relatively straightforward and quick-paced manner (that is, you are in early labor, experiencing regular contractions, within five to seven hours after your waters have broken), you will have a hospital experience much like those of women whose labors begin with contractions. In most studies of PROM, around 70 to 75 percent of women go into spontaneous labor within 24 hours and 85 percent within 48 hours. Knowing that statistics are on your side may help you feel more relaxed about this situation.

If, however, you do not start to feel contractions soon after your waters break or five or more hours pass without the advent of regular contractions, you are likely to face considerable pressure to "do something" about this. The pressure is motivated by a belief in obstetrical circles that "prolonged rupture of the membranes" can result in life-threatening infections for mother, baby, or both. The catch is that no one can precisely define *prolonged*. This is an area where science and obstetrical practice are not entirely in sync. The many studies that have been done of prolonged rupture of the membranes have produced no evidence that induction reduces rates of infection in otherwise healthy and group-B-strep-negative mothers and babies (Hannah et al., 1996; Centers for Disease Control and Prevention, 2002; Mozurkewich, 2006).

Women who have tested positive for group B strep must consider the pros and cons of induction versus waiting more carefully than those who have tested negative. There have been few studies in which group-B-strep-positive women with ruptured membranes have been allowed to begin active labor spontaneously. We just do not know whether, or in what situations, group B strep poses a real risk to infants in the womb. As researchers Amy Marowitz and Robin Jordan (2007, p. 199) conclude, "Certainty regarding optimal management remains elusive." The worry is that the longer the baby is unprotected by the bag of waters, the more risk the strep may pose to the baby. Because in very rare cases a baby dies from group B strep, most practitioners are very cautious.

An excellent source of information that summarizes the current science about deciding whether to induce when your water breaks after you have reached 37 weeks of pregnancy and about the specific situation for women who test positive for group B strep is located on the Evidence-Based Birth website. Here are the URLs for specific, relevant pages: evidencebasedbirth.com/evidence-inducing-labor-water-breaks-term and evidencebasedbirth.com/groupbstrep.

If you have tested positive for group B strep, I recommend that you research your options and take steps to minimize group B strep in your vagina in the last weeks of your pregnancy. Natural-leaning doctors recommend eating fermented foods. After dietary changes, some group-B-strep-positive women have retested as negative. You might also decide to accept the routine antibiotic treatment for group B strep without accepting other interventions, such as induction or augmentation with Pitocin.

Vaginal Exams and PROM

There is extremely strong evidence that reducing the number of vaginal exams after the bag of waters has broken reduces the rates of infection in all women, regardless of group-B-strep status (Soper et al., 1996; Marowitz & Jordan, 2007). Let's look at this more closely. The reason that we think vaginal exams increase rates of maternal infection is that there are always bacteria living in our vaginas. But, normally, the bacteria at the lower end of the vaginal canal do not move upward toward the cervix. In fact, vaginal secretions (and amniotic fluid, when your water has broken) flow downward, not upward. But inserting anything into the vagina, such as a finger or a penis, gives that bacteria a free ride upward. This effect is clearly demonstrated in the statistics below:

If a woman receives 3 to 4 vaginal exams after her waters have broken, her chance of uterine infection is twice that of women who do not receive vaginal exams.

If a woman receives 7 to 8 vaginal exams, those odds rise to 3.8 times.

And if a woman receives more than 8 vaginal exams, she has five times the chance of developing a uterine infection (Dekker, 2017).

It's also useful to know that having more vaginal exams in the last weeks of pregnancy increases the chance that you will experience PROM in the first place (Lenihan, 1984). Vaginal exams at the end of pregnancy do not give us any information that helps us predict anything at all, so declining late-pregnancy vaginal exams is a good idea for virtually all women.

Despite the strong evidence, even doctors and nurses who are aware of the risks of vaginal exams seem to have difficulty with the hands-off approach. In one labor I attended, the nurse advised my client that she should not have "too many" vaginal exams since her waters had broken. Ironically, the nurse delivered this advice as she had her gloved fingers inside my client's vagina.

On the one hand, you are unlikely to face this scenario. You have a greater than 75 percent chance that you will either begin having contractions or go into active labor soon after your waters break. On the other hand, beginning active labor with a ruptured bag of waters is one of the most common situations that result in medical interventions and unnecessary C-sections, so it is an excellent idea to have a plan for this possibility. Read on to learn why an ounce of prevention is worth a pound of cure in this situation.

What Usually Happens When There Is No Plan in Place

When a woman's bag of waters breaks before contractions begin, catching her and her partner off guard, they may make decisions based on fear rather than knowledge. Heavily influenced by a nurse's or doctor's use of the chilling words *possible life-threatening infection*, clients agree to an induction. Induction with synthetic oxytocin (Pitocin) or misoprostol (Cytotec) typically leads to stronger, harder, and longer contractions than the woman would experience naturally. Some women manage to labor on Pitocin without needing an epidural, but the majority opt for pharmaceutical relief from the pain. These synthetic hormones mimic the ones our bodies make, but they do not prompt our bodies to release endorphins or decrease the production of adrenaline.

Induction appears to be related to an increased risk of cesarean, compared to what is called "expectant management" (which means waiting for labor to begin on its own). Although some studies report only a slightly elevated or even slightly decreased cesarean rate in such cases, several large studies have found that early induction after the spontaneous rupture of the membranes "tripled or quadrupled the chances of

C-section" (Goer, 1999, p. 231). In the first large-scale study of PROM to be completed using testing and treatment for group B strep, the difference was stark: women who were induced had a five times greater chance of ending with a cesarean than did women who waited for labor to begin (Pintucci et al., 2014).

Why do women in this situation so often end up in the surgery room? Because of the heightened attention to fever in their labors combined with the high rate of epidurals. Fever can be caused by an epidural, but it is also the first and best indication of an infection. When women whose membranes have been ruptured for any length of time develop a fever, the idea of a C-section starts to percolate. The medical team worries that any infection the mother may have will immediately be transmitted to the baby because the baby has lost her protective bag of waters. They also worry about an infection developing inside the uterus, which would be far more serious than an infection elsewhere.

Your care providers may say they have no way of knowing whether your temperature is due to an infection (solution: emergency cesarean) or if you have an epidural, whether it is simply due to the epidural (solution: keep on laboring as you are). At this point, it is impossible for most women, partners, and their caregivers to avoid a C-section. There is almost no way to determine the cause of the fever until after the birth, which is obviously too late. Many thousands of unnecessary C-sections are performed in this scenario.

How to Avoid a Cesarean

The key is to avoid induction and, after that, an epidural. If you develop a fever in the absence of an epidural, you will know that the fever is likely due to an infection. You will have to make the tough choices this situation requires, but you will never have to second-guess whether an epidural caused the fever.

Before Your Waters Break:
The "Special Exception" Caregiver Clause

Once your waters break, you may feel at the mercy of your hospital or caregiver's protocol unless you have planned ahead. If you have thought through this scenario and included your wishes in your birth plan, you will be better equipped to resist any pressure to use pharmaceutical drugs to speed up your labor. Before you face this situation, you can

• prepare your plan in case your waters break before contractions begin; and

• get your doctor or midwife to agree with your plan.

Whether you are working with a midwife, a family doctor, or an obstetrician, there is a high likelihood that your prenatal caregiver will not be attending your baby's birth. The birth attendant may be whoever is on call the day you deliver. So it may not seem to make much sense to get your medical caregiver on board with your plan.

However, the statement "My midwife/doctor supports my plan" can be powerful. I have seen this sentence turn situations around instantly. "Oh?" said one nurse. "I'm not used to that, but if they say so. . . ." Other nurses may be irked. "Well, your doctor isn't here right now," they may retort. Yet the fact that you have gotten "permission" from your caregiver means that the staff cannot pretend that there is no choice.

At some point in your pregnancy, before introducing your birth plan, discuss with your caregiver the possibility that your membranes will rupture before contractions begin. Ask how he would handle the situation. You are most interested in reaching agreement about two issues, so that you can include these items on your birth plan with your caregiver's support:

1. Waiting for contractions to begin naturally, without induction

2. Avoiding unnecessary vaginal exams

Asking, "What do you generally advise women to do if their waters break before contractions begin?" is a good way to start. If the caregiver's response dovetails with your desires, great! You're all set.

But, if your doctor or midwife talks about wanting "to see you go into labor/have the baby within *X* hours," take a deep breath. Find your most reasonable, accommodating, peaceful voice. I recommend that you start this conversation by reiterating not only how important natural childbirth is to you but why it is important to you. You might say you believe that natural birth will be better for your health and your baby's, but avoid any medical arguments. Your demonstration of personal commitment, more than your medical knowledge, will likely be the make-it-or-break-it factor when you are dealing with a caregiver who disagrees with you. You are never going to convince a caregiver who has developed a different style of handling childbirth that you are right. You can, however, convince your caregiver that you deeply desire something different and that his support matters to you.

Your caregiver might say something like, "Well, I see that you are very committed to natural childbirth, but I can't in good conscience let you go more than twenty-four hours without recommending induction. I would be putting you at risk for infection." Or, he might avoid the topic by saying, "Let's just handle that if it comes up. There's no use worrying unnecessarily now." At worst, the practitioner will feel so defensive that he goes on the attack, telling you that you care more about your birth experience than the health of your baby.

In response to any of these, I recommend that you persevere with a direct request. "Certainly, my most important objective is a healthy baby. Your support for our plan would give me peace of mind. If I develop a fever or the baby isn't doing well, I will be willing to reconsider. But if I do not get a fever and the baby is doing fine, I would really appreciate your support to go forty-eight hours before we talk about induction. And since I'm planning to go natural, I'd also like to avoid vaginal exams until I get close to the end of labor, again assuming that I don't have a fever and the baby is doing well." Forty-eight hours is the amount of time that the researchers in the 2014 Pintucci study used before women in their study were induced, so it is the amount of waiting time for which we have recent evidence.

If there seems to be some mutual understanding with your caregiver, you can press further. You can also say that you'd rather visit the caregiver's office than the hospital, after your waters break, if it is necessary to determine whether the umbilical cord has prolapsed. A prolapsed cord means that the umbilical cord has slipped below the baby and in the absence of amniotic fluid to float everything in the womb, could get compressed. Most caregivers want to check on this possibility if a woman's waters break early in labor. It's much better to go to the office, if possible, than the hospital. The hospital staff would likely try to convince you to check in and stay, yet you may have many hours ahead of you without contractions. It's much easier to walk out of your caregiver's office than hospital triage, the place where women in labor usually go to be examined before they are admitted. See pages 93 to 94 for Allison's story about leaving the hospital in this situation.

I have found that many caregivers, though certainly not all, will give special permission for individual patients' unorthodox choices. Your caregiver might say to you, "I usually like to see women deliver within twelve hours of membrane rupture, but I'll make an exception for you."

If your caregiver is put off by your request, at least you know what you are dealing with ahead of time. With that information, you can make choices. You may still decide to go ahead with your own plan, especially if it is likely that you will have a different caregiver at the time of delivery.

Before Active Labor Begins

When your waters break, don't look at the clock. I'm including this piece of advice because it has worked for some women who genuinely did not know the time their membranes ruptured. Unfortunately, most of us are so surrounded by clocks that they are impossible to avoid. But you should see the nurses desperately try to pin down a woman who says, "I don't know what time exactly."

Give yourself twenty-four to forty-eight hours without accepting or if you can avoid it, even considering intervention. If a medical professional has said to you, "If things don't get going by X o'clock, we'll have to consider inducing," you are likely to feel like a watched pot. Your mind becomes a spectator of your own body, and this has the horrible consequence of slowing down your labor. How do you circumvent this problem? By assigning your support team to talk to the medical professionals, so your mind does not need to get involved, and by keeping a strong commitment to giving your body the time it needs to adjust to labor.

Your doctor's or hospital's recommendations are just that: recommendations. Each hospital has a different clock. The typical twenty-four-hour wait for induction developed as a rule of thumb in the 1960s. It has withstood neither the test of time nor the test of scientific scrutiny. Some hospital protocols stipulate that women can wait eight hours, others twelve, and still others twenty-four or forty-eight to go into labor spontaneously before doctors are supposed to recommend induction. Protocols vary widely.

There are two ways that you are likely to hear the phrase "twenty-four hours" (or, if you are at a progressive hospital, "forty-eight hours") in relation to ruptured membranes. On the one hand, many caregivers believe that "the baby must be born within twenty-four hours" of the rupture. On the other hand, most studies of prelabor ROM allow women to go a full twenty-four hours before their labors are *induced*, which means that their babies are definitely not born within twenty-four hours of the waters breaking.

Even within the same hospital, personnel interpret protocols very differently. The differences can be frustrating if you don't have a strong sense of what *you* want. Here is a good example of the variety of opinions you can encounter:

> *My client Suzy started off her hospital experience in triage, two hours after her membranes had ruptured, with a doctor who recommended immediate induction. When she asked for more time to decide, we found ourselves in a hospital room with a nurse who talked as though there was absolutely no way around induction. According to her, if labor didn't start within a few hours, Suzy "must" be induced. Then, the doctor who had provided Suzy's prenatal care gave us carte blanche to continue with natural labor as long as we desired, provided Suzy didn't spike a fever. Her doctor arranged for us to be assigned a new nurse. Our next nurse was supportive of waiting, and several pleasant hours went by without a fuss. Unfortunately, there was a shift change before Suzy gave birth. Our next nurse agreed that it was Suzy's choice but strongly pushed induction along with an epidural.*

Suzy did manage to avoid an induction. So don't take your caregiver's recommendations as rules, especially if your caregiver is recommending induction without allowing at least twenty-four to forty-eight hours for contractions to begin spontaneously. Evidence exists that even seventy-two hours without induction is safe (Shalev et al., 1995), so "immediate induction" is not supported by evidence without other risk factors being present.

Stay at home or visit your caregiver's office. The easiest way to avoid the pressures of hospital protocols is to stay at home (Bridget and Eric's story on pages 146 to 147 and Shannon and Kevin's story in Chapter Fifteen exemplify how helpful staying home can be). Do check the color of your amniotic fluid, however. If it is clear, you might consult with your doula or caregiver by phone and then just go about your business (refer to pages 141 to 143 for ideas on how to spend your time in early labor). If the amniotic fluid is not clear and especially if it is dark-colored (green, gray, or brown), call your care provider immediately, go to the hospital, or both, because dark amniotic fluid may be a sign that your baby is in distress.

Because your caregiver is likely to want to check for the position of the umbilical cord and listen to the baby's heart rate, it is helpful to have an agreement that you will go to her office rather than the hospital for this exam. If your waters break at night, you may have no choice but to go to the hospital. Bring your partner, a friend, or your doula with you. Be prepared to politely decline being admitted once you know that the umbilical cord and baby are in good position.

Ideally, the caregiver will make this determination by checking your baby's heart rate, not by giving you a vaginal exam. Since vaginal exams increase the chances of infection when the waters are broken, be politely insistent on this point!

Go back home! If you have gone to the hospital to get checked and either contractions have not kicked in or you are still in early labor, you will often get sent home. If the triage staff want to keep you, insist that you want to go home. If home is too far away, tell them you would like to go to a restaurant or a hotel for a few hours. I once worked with a woman whose waters broke at 2 a.m. Her doctor had told her to go straight to the hospital if her waters broke. Yet, once she had been checked, the staff suggested that she go home. Unfortunately, it took three hours to get discharged. Since her home was forty-five minutes away, she and her husband rented a hotel room a few blocks from the hospital and spent about four hours watching movies and napping. Once you are in the hospital, sometimes you have to be pushy—or just get up to leave—to make a discharge happen. Because your case is not an emergency, you may land at the bottom of the staff's priorities.

Drink a lot of water. Your body will continue making amniotic fluid and trying to fill the nonexistent water bag around the baby. You need a lot of water.

Once Active Labor Begins

Continue to ignore the clock. Hurray! You are in active labor. Proceed to the next chapter for tips.

If at any time your midwife, doctor, or nurse acts as though you are still on a clock (by insisting, for example, that you must deliver your baby within twenty-four hours of your waters' breaking or they will "do something" like order a Pitocin drip), ask her to support your plan to put off intervention unless you develop a fever or there is strong evidence of fetal distress. Better yet, make sure during pregnancy that your partner is ready for this particular conversation.

Keep drinking water and avoid a fever-causing epidural. Tips for avoiding an epidural are included in the next chapters. You're on your way!

Transition to the Hospital

"Let's go, honey," someone says. And it feels right. You try to pick up your bag by the front door, but a contraction hits you just as you bend over. You lean against the wall and breathe through it while your partner races around gathering last-minute items. As soon as the contraction is over, you open the door and walk outside. You leave the bag sitting on the floor. You know that if you do not get moving you will never make it to the car.

Isabelle Yingling, a doula and Bradley childbirth-preparation instructor from Ottawa, tells couples that if you can get from your house to the car in less than ten minutes, you are going to the hospital too early.

The car ride to the hospital can be the worst part of a labor experience. I have knelt in the back seat with women as they struggled through intense contractions on bumpy roads. Anything that jars your body during a contraction makes the pain worse. I have also known many women who went to the hospital and were advised to go back home, but who insisted on checking into the hospital because they could not bear the thought of two more car rides during labor.

If you live more than half an hour from your hospital, consider alternative possibilities. Is a hotel nearby? Does a friend or relative live near the hospital? You might consider going to one of these places in early labor so that your transition to the hospital in active labor won't be so painful.

Even if your car ride is under thirty minutes, these minutes are likely to be difficult for you. The good news is that by traveling in a car during active labor, instead of early labor, you are increasing your chances of delivering a healthy baby safely and naturally. Concentrating on the reasons why you have chosen your course of action will help you feel strong and empowered even through the bumps. Bring along a friend who can focus on your needs during the ride, even if this person is not invited to attend the birth.

Triage (Check-in)

Most hospitals, though not all, require laboring women to check in at "triage." This is where someone determines the status of your labor and whether to admit you. Some hospitals ask you to come in during your third trimester to fill out paperwork that will speed up the check-in process. Even if you do this, there usually are absurd amounts of questions to answer and papers to fill out in triage. Ideally, you will be so far into your labor that the nurses will do everything fast to get you into a birthing room and then direct most of their questions at your support people. A woman in San Francisco writes that "I arrived at the hospital at 9 centimeters after thirty-nine hours of labor. I was moaning like a cow. The attending nurse-midwife came around the corner as I exited the elevator and smiled when she said, 'Now there's a sound we don't hear very often! The sound of a natural childbirth.'" This woman was able to skip triage altogether and check into her birthing room directly.

Because you will be in active labor, your support person should be prepared to do as much of the talking and paperwork as possible. Although the staff are supposed to get answers from you, if they can, it is much easier to have your support person answer questions and then say, "Is that right?" All you have to do is nod your head. Make sure your support person knows the answers to questions about your medical history, such as these:

• Are you allergic to any medications? (You will probably be asked this question at least ten times before your baby is born!)

• Have you had high blood pressure during your pregnancy?

• Are you on any medications now? If so, which? When was your last dose?

If there have been any complications during your pregnancy or if you have any specific health conditions that affect pregnancy (such as diabetes, high blood pressure, or epilepsy), please make sure that your support person knows the details of these conditions intimately. Write them down and bring a cheat sheet with you to the hospital.

I was a doula for one couple who had achieved pregnancy through in-vitro fertilization (IVF). It is common for women who undergo IVF to take prescription drugs during pregnancy. In this case, she was prescribed the drug heparin and a daily aspirin. She discontinued both of these drugs several weeks before her due date. In the twenty-four hours that she was in the hospital, she was asked at least twenty times about what drugs she had taken and what dates she discontinued them. Each new nurse, doctor, and intern repeated the questions as they read over her chart. I believe it would have eased her labor considerably if her husband had been prepared to answer most of these questions.

Sometimes, support people feel that they are stepping on a mother's toes by answering questions like "What is your birth date?" and "How far apart are contractions now?" Agree beforehand that even if you are able to answer, your support person is going to take the leading role.

Know that the triage staff are not your birth team. The nurses and doctors here are likely not the nurses and doctors who work on the labor-and-delivery floor. So save your team-building efforts for the staff who will be with you in the hours ahead.

A nurse or a doctor will ask you questions about how your labor began, how long it has been going on, and so on. He will go over any unusual points in your medical chart. Then he will listen to the baby's heartbeat and will likely hook you up to an external fetal monitor to get a "strip." This strip (usually ten to twenty-five minutes of recording) shows the triage staff the pattern of the baby's heartbeat and measures the intensity of your contractions. The nurse or doctor will also want to do a vaginal exam.

Initial Vaginal Exam

Before you arrive at the hospital, know whether or not, and under which conditions, you wish to have vaginal exams.

Most women arrive eager to know their magic number. You will probably be hoping the triage nurse will reach in, smile, and say, "Congratulations! You're fully dilated!" I hope this is what happens to you. It's much more likely, however, that you will get a number in the 2-to-5 range. Be forewarned that you are likely to feel some disappointment. In all my experience, I have met only a handful of women who did not find the initial vaginal exam at least a little discouraging. We almost all hope for a bigger number than we get.

At the initial vaginal exam, you can ask for any other information the doctor or nurse has gleaned. For instance, is the baby positioned high or low? Did the practitioner feel whether the head was well applied to the cervix and in a good position? Many nurses don't share this information unless they are asked directly.

A final note about vaginal exams: Measuring dilation is not a precise science. Every person who measures a cervix does so with fingers, not with a ruler. It is therefore in your best interest to have the same person do all your vaginal exams. There is nothing more frustrating that having a nurse tell you that you are 6 centimeters dilated and then having a doctor come in an hour later and tell you that you are at 5.

If your bag of waters is not broken and you do not have objections to vaginal exams, I recommend that you request a second vaginal exam as soon as you move from triage to your room. Your nurse is likely to tell you that nothing much will have changed since your exam in triage. But your objective is to start off with a measurement by this nurse, with her fingers. The only exception to this would be if you are admitted close to a change of shift, in which case you will be getting a new nurse soon anyway.

If You Do Not Want to Have a Vaginal Exam

There are situations in which women should avoid exams. If your waters have broken, you are well advised to avoid all vaginal exams. (Try to get your doctor to agree to this plan in advance; see pages 158 to 159.) Some survivors of sexual abuse find vaginal exams so traumatic that their labors are significantly and negatively affected by them. Finally, some women just do not want to know how dilated they are. They are experiencing their labor in their bodies, and external information feels wrong.

Here is the triage nurse's likely reaction to your request not to do a vaginal exam: "If I don't do an exam, I can't tell where you are in labor. I can't admit you if I don't know whether you're in active labor." Your support person can answer, "We'd really like to wait to have a vaginal exam. Could you please evaluate her labor based on all the other evidence?" The nurse can then consider how intense the contractions appear, how long they last, how close together they are, how long you have been in labor, whether your waters have broken, and how you are breathing and behaving. In short, if the triage nurse can't tell that you are in labor without doing an internal exam, you may still be in early labor.

Congratulations! You're in the hospital. You are minutes or hours or perhaps a day away from seeing your baby.

chapter 9

ACTIVE LABOR: TAKING YOUR TIME

"W E'D LIKE TO WAIT AN HOUR."
These words should be at the tip of your and your support person's tongue at all times. In response to virtually any suggestion for intervening in labor, say, "We'd like to wait an hour." If you remember nothing else, remember to say, "We'd like to wait an hour."

In hospitals, people work on schedules that are determined by many important considerations. Normally, we respect these schedules. When we visit the hospital for an X-ray or a biopsy, we are not in the habit of saying, "I'd like to wait an hour." If we accompany a family member to the emergency room and wait for hours, we might be annoyed, but we rarely press our own schedule on the hospital. However, labor is different.

Your body and your baby will birth best at their own pace. Your baby has little regard for whether the doctor is about to leave your floor for a surgery; your uterus does not care whether the woman next door is about to deliver. Your pace is your pace.

Some interventions in your labor are offered because of the hospital's schedule. Examples include fetal heart monitoring on a schedule or a nurse arriving just minutes after a woman has fallen asleep to introduce herself because the nurse has just started her shift. Other interventions are offered because the staff are concerned about your particular labor.

Unless there is a true emergency, delaying procedures is often a good decision for women who want to give birth naturally. And there is no danger in using the sentence "We'd like to wait an hour," even in a crisis. If there is an emergency, you will know it. In an urgent situation, events will be out of your control. If you say, "We'd like to wait an hour," the hospital staff will not even hear you. You and your caregivers will make the best decisions that you can make in a crisis.

By contrast, if your situation is not an emergency, you have time to think, consider, react, plan, try other options. If you don't know whether the situation you are in is truly an emergency, it is not an emergency. You have time. In fact, you probably have an hour.

Some readers of the first edition of this book objected to this advice. They thought it might set women up to feel adversarial with hospital staff and create an "us-against-them" feeling. Ironically, I give this advice precisely because I hope to protect the positive relationship a birthing woman and her team develop with hospital staff. To be clear, there are many, many care providers who do not offer unnecessary interventions during most labors. You may not need this tool at all! In my town, this is probably true at about 15 to 20 percent of uncomplicated births that I attend as a doula.

If no interventions are offered, you won't have to say this phrase; but if an intervention is offered that you don't really want, this phrase can be extremely helpful. I have found that refusing the intervention or arguing about whether the intervention is warranted creates much worse discord than asking for more time. The alternatives, as I see them, are to:

- Acquiesce with the suggested intervention, even if you don't really want it at that time.

- Refuse the suggested intervention.

- Argue with the staff and try to convince them that their suggestion is not correct.

- Get yourself more time.

I think that, given the alternatives, getting more time for your body do its work on its own is your best option—and also the option most likely to foster goodwill with the staff without accepting an unnecessary intervention.

Here are some situations in which the handy sentence "We'd like to wait an hour" works magic. Try it if your nurse, midwife, or doctor wants to:

• perform a vaginal exam;

• hook you up to an external fetal monitor for a "strip;"

• hook you up to an external fetal monitor for the duration of labor;

• break your bag of waters (to check on the baby, to speed up your labor, or both);

• give you Pitocin to strengthen your contractions;

• put an internal fetal monitor on the baby;

• give you pain-relieving drugs; or

• do a C-section.

When you say, "We'd like to wait an hour," your nurse, doctor, or midwife will probably try to convince you to comply. Try to concentrate on what you want—time for your body to give birth—rather than on what you are trying to avoid. Try the broken-record approach. Think of how many different ways you can say the same thing: "We'd like to wait an hour." The conversation might sound like this:

Midwife/doctor/nurse: I'd like to do *X,* just to be sure.

Your support person: We'd like to wait an hour before we do that.

Midwife/doctor/nurse: Well, I'd really like to know a bit more about what's going on.

Your support person: Well, you know Jasmine really, really wants a natural birth. It's extremely important to her. We'd like more time to labor. It's just so important to her to do everything possible to have a natural birth.

Midwife/doctor/nurse: I just want to make sure the baby is doing OK. That's more important than what kind of birth she has.

Your support person: Still, natural birth is really important to us, and it sounds like the baby is not in danger right this minute. We'd like to wait an hour.

Midwife/doctor/nurse: Well, I don't really want to wait longer than an hour, and I can't guarantee that I'll be back within an hour to do this, so I'd really rather do it now. [*Note: The caregiver has just provided a golden piece of information: This is not an emergency situation. Part of the reason for the push is her schedule. It's OK to wait an hour.*]

Your support person: I appreciate your concern. Since we're doing so well right now [*or* Since we're trying to get back into a good labor pattern], I think waiting an hour is the best thing to do right now.

This support person successfully redirects the conversation and everyone's attention to the woman's need for support in her natural labor.

Avoiding Confrontation

Saying what you want can feel confrontational. If you balk at a suggestion in a way that seems accusatory, the person is likely to fight back. But if you just assert what you want, most caregivers will avoid escalating the situation into a confrontation. They, like you, do not want to be the bad guy. By sticking with what you want rather than questioning your caregivers' expertise, you will succeed surprisingly often.

Asking for a time extension is often a good way to walk this fine line. Think about high school or college. If you told your teacher that you didn't want to do a particular assignment, the teacher would likely refuse your request to skip it. But if you explained to your teacher why doing the assignment right now was impossible—you had a championship soccer game that evening, or you were to be the bridesmaid in your sister's wedding that weekend—and suggested that you could do the assignment later, your teacher would be much more likely to acquiesce.

Here are two more sample dialogues to show you how this works:

Scenario 1. Your nurse, midwife, or doctor says, "I'd like to perform a vaginal exam now."

Your supporter first says what you want and then asks for a time extension: "She is doing really well in this position. I don't want her to get discouraged by a number right now, when we're doing so well. Could we wait an hour before checking again?"

Scenario 2. Your nurse, midwife, or doctor says, "I'd like to hook you up to an external fetal monitor for a strip."

Your supporter says, "She was just about to use the toilet and then try the shower. We could do that strip in an hour." In this case, your supporter might also ask to have the baby's heart rate checked in some other way: "I've heard of some other device that can get the baby's heart rate. Do you have one of those handheld kinds?" If no handheld device is available, your supporter might offer to hold the heart rate monitor on your belly while you are standing, for a quick check. You might agree to a longer monitoring later.

Distinguishing Emergencies from Nonemergencies

Though you will know a true emergency if it happens, you won't necessarily recognize a nonemergency. Laboring mothers and their support teams often feel as though they are experiencing an emergency even when they are not. Much of today's medicine is about evaluating risk, so even normal labors are continuously assessed as potentially hazardous. Your labor might be progressing perfectly, but the language of danger that is often spoken at hospitals might make you fear that you or your baby is in trouble. You may have exceptional caregivers who take care to speak calmly and respectfully with all laboring women, so this may not apply to your particular hospital or caregiver. But the phenomenon is widespread enough that most women should know how to safeguard their own feelings of peace.

Though you may look to the hospital staff members for reassurance and help in remaining calm, in fact, this is not their primary role. Excellent as they may be at caring for patients, physically and emotionally, labor-and-delivery nurses must give physical tests priority over reassurance. You have hired them to monitor the physical progress of your labor and uncover potential problems. They are experts at this job.

Often, what they find is ambiguous: perhaps there is a developing problem; perhaps there is not. They are often, but not necessarily, skilled at delivering their findings in words that reassure us.

That caregivers really have a variety of levels of skill in "bedside manner" is not news. Some midwives, medical residents, obstetricians, anesthesiologists, and pediatricians have excellent empathy and communication skills. I find that residents are often the most rushed, exhausted, and worried about making a mistake. (Though even among residents, this varies widely; some are amazing!) I am not trying to make a blanket statement about birth professionals. I am just reminding you that their *primary job* is to keep your body and your baby safe, which includes constantly thinking about possible complications that could arise. They may or may not be able to communicate about those "possible complications" well.

But your job is *not* to think about possible complications. Because *you* produce the hormones that affect your labor, you must take responsibility for remaining calm. You cannot outsource this to your doctor or midwife or nurses. Be prepared to face possible emergency language with equanimity. In pregnancy, you can train yourself to reach a tranquil state with ease. Any number of methods can help: childbirth-preparation programs, yoga classes, relaxing hot baths, meditation, mindfulness practices, and massage, to name a few. Even if you face a true emergency in the hospital, in which case there will be no possibility of waiting an hour for nature to take its course, making decisions calmly will feel better than making them in a panic.

You will know you're facing an emergency if you say that you would like to wait an hour and your caregivers look at you as if you were crazy or tell you that they are trying to save your baby's life or your own. In many emergencies, caregivers don't even bother answering. They are concentrating on the work at hand.

But there are clues you and your supporters can pursue to confirm that there is indeed time for nature's work. Here are some common scenarios that indicate a nonemergency:

• A staff member tells you that you should take advantage of an opportunity now because the doctor/anesthesiologist/nurse may not be available an hour from now when you might want the intervention.

- The doctor/midwife/nurse tells you that this intervention isn't necessary, but that she would like to get more information. This is especially likely when the suggestion is to break the bag of waters. If the goal is simply more information, there is no emergency right now. You might ask, "How else could we get more information?" or, "We'd like to wait an hour."

- Your caregiver takes time to argue that the suggested procedure is a good idea. In an emergency, there would be no time for lengthy explanations.

- Your doctor/midwife/nurse tells you that yes, you *could* wait, but she doesn't advise it. Follow-up questions, probably by your partner if you are in active labor, should help you understand the situation better.

Natural Labor versus Institutional Needs

I was a doula for a couple in Toronto who desired a natural birth. Because the mother, Maria, had a number of health problems, her doctor asked her to go to the hospital right away if her waters broke before she could feel contractions. Her labor did begin this way, so we arrived at the hospital in very early labor. The doctor on call and our first two nurses insisted that she would have to be given Pitocin immediately to get labor going. We kept asking for deferrals. The nurses were not happy with our requests and kept telling us that we had "no choice."

After about three hours, the nurse again insisted that Maria should be started on a Pitocin intravenous drip, and we again asked to defer for an hour. The nurse told Maria, evidently to scare her into accepting the IV, "Right now you're not in active labor. If you're not on Pitocin or in active labor, I can't keep you on the labor-and-delivery floor. I'll have to send you to the antenatal floor.* And then when you go into labor, there's no guarantee that there will be a room here for you. We're very busy. You might not get a room when you need one. And you'll have to share a room on the antenatal floor. So it won't be so nice for you."

---

* *The antenatal floor is for pregnant women who are hospitalized for complications.*

She delivered this warning in an ominous voice. We were all cowed. But as soon as she left the room I felt a rise of joy and laughter. "Well," I said. "That's it. Now we know why they're pushing the Pitocin so hard."

"What about how there might not be a room for me later?" Maria asked.

"When you are in active labor, they will find a place for you to have your baby," I said. With the information the nurse had given us in her tirade, we were able to fend off the Pitocin completely. We moved to the antenatal floor. Eventually, when Maria went into active labor, we were reassigned to the labor-and-delivery floor without a problem. The nurses on the antenatal floor made sure that we got a birthing room very quickly. They did not relish the idea of a full-blown labor (much less delivery) on their floor.

If you have spent a lot of time in hospitals, you know that hospital staff people move at their own pace. Doctors and nurses may disappear from your room for long stretches of time. Then, when they reappear, they are ready for brisk action. Keeping the sentence "We'd like to wait an hour" ready at all times is your best defense against unnecessary intervention.

chapter 10

ACTIVE LABOR: COPING WITH MEANINGFUL PAIN

"T HE BEST MOMENTS [OF LIFE] usually occur when a person's body or mind is stretched to its limits in a voluntary effort to accomplish something difficult and worthwhile," observes creativity expert Mihaly Csikszentmihalyi (2008, p. 3). And nothing is going to stretch your body and your mind more than labor. Labor is hard. It is really, really, really hard.

In this chapter, we will focus on how to handle the pain of labor. The time-tested techniques that our great-grandmothers used are numerous. If one does not work, you can try another. Techniques include conscious relaxation, visualization, breathing, physical movement (changing positions), using water, eating for energy, Rebozo techniques, letting your emotions flow freely, and hearing words of reassurance. When you feel pain in your back, you can also try counterpressure and hip squeezing to relieve pain.

Make sure that your birth team is adequately prepared to help you with all these techniques. If you have hired a doula, talk with her in-depth about your preferences. Ask her to demonstrate her techniques (such as back pressure, massage, and vocal coaching) while you are pregnant. You should feel calmer knowing exactly what kind of support you can expect.

If your spouse, a friend, or a relative will be your primary labor coach, be sure to practice pain-relieving techniques with that person. The two of you shouldn't just read books about birth. Your companion must learn to respond to your physical cues, such as changes in your breathing or tension in your face or body, and should have well-practiced words of endearment to offer when you need them (see "The Power of 'I Love You': A Note For Partners" on page 191 and "Using Words of Encouragement," page 192). You need confidence that your primary coach will respond as you want in your moments of greatest fear or overwhelming pain, and you will gain that confidence only by practicing labor management techniques together. As with learning a foreign language, the two of you have to practice over and over again to make your responses second nature.

> There are two ways of meeting difficulties.
> You alter the difficulty, or you alter yourself to meet them.
>
> **— PHYLLIS BOTTOME**
>
> Everything in life that we really accept undergoes a change.
>
> **— KATHERINE MANSFIELD**

Relaxation

The only way I know to get through labor pain is to surrender to it. *Achieving* surrender is the hard part. When you feel overwhelmed by contractions, you have not yet surrendered. You are in pre-surrender. A miracle happens in the instant that you yield. Labor stops feeling so hard. You stop feeling overwhelmed. As soon as you accept that labor is overwhelming, it ceases to be so. Relaxing during painful contractions changes the feeling of those contractions. This is just one of life's paradoxes.

Getting through the worst labor pain may be your deepest physical challenge as a woman. Few physical challenges that we can choose voluntarily equal the sensations of labor. Some of us may have undertaken serious challenges, such as hiking long distances with a heavy backpack, going to boot camp, doing strenuous garden or farm work, or training for a sport. Otherwise, serious physical challenges are usually out of our control and are associated with enormous fear, such as pain from a car accident or of an illness like cancer. Birth and physical achievements are different from disease in that the pain of birth or exertion does not signal a problem. As childbirth expert Penny Simkin says, birth pain is different from suffering. Birth is less like a car accident and much more like the experience of athletes who must find in themselves an extra bit of strength to end a marathon with a sprint. You, like the marathon runner, will learn about your own depths. You will find a "flow" from a reservoir of seemingly divine strength, determination, and endurance.

Yet, before you find the flow, you are likely to experience overwhelming pain. Some women never experience unmanageable pain in their labors, but most do at some point. For many women, this point coincides with transition, the final cervical opening from 8 to 10 centimeters. In a first labor, using muscles never before tested, your uterus has stretched far beyond what it has ever done before just to get to 7 centimeters. But it can't stop there. It—and you—must keep going. The last centimeters require more strength, more effort from your muscles (physical, mental, emotional, and spiritual muscles) than you have ever given to anything before.

For some women, this feeling of being overwhelmed occurs earlier in labor. Perhaps you have been laboring for many, many hours, and you are bone-tired. Or the pain at 6 centimeters is really the worst you ever imagined, and now you are absolutely terrified of what will come next. If this feeling arises before 7 centimeters of dilation, this very well could be the worst pain of your labor. I have worked with many women who experienced intense pain at 5 to 6 centimeters as their bodies prepared to undergo a rapid acceleration of labor. Later, they said this was the worst part of labor.

The crucible of extended pain tests a woman's resolve to have a natural birth. Did you mean that you wanted a natural birth as long as it wasn't too difficult? As long as you had a relatively easy labor and the contractions never got too overwhelming? Or did you mean you wanted to scrape the bottom of your soul for the last remaining shards of determination? Some women have natural births only because they deliver so fast that there is no time for medical intervention. And other women have easy contractions that never test their mettle. All of us wish we fell into these categories, but the fact is that most of us do not.

Whether a feeling of doubt arises at 3 or 9 centimeters, you will feel frustrated, overwhelmed, flooded, out of control—in a word: panicked.

You doubt that you can do this for one minute longer. For even a second longer. The next contraction may just kill you. Even if you ordered an epidural now, you're not sure you could last the half hour it generally takes to get it started.

Relax. Take a deep breath.

At this point, you have reached the climax of the thinking mind's journey in labor. As long as you are thinking about how labor feels, you are unconsciously comparing it to what you expected or what you think may lie ahead. Saying goodbye to your thinking mind is difficult for many of us, especially those of us who use our brains to make a living. We pride ourselves on how well we think. We enjoy feeling competent and in control. Our culture does not give us many lessons in the value of surrendering to forces larger than our own logic.

This is the time you need your coach to be more focused, calm, and reassuring than ever before. You need reminders from your coaches and professional helpers to relax, take a deep breath, and focus on just this moment. You need to hear no panic in their voices. If you have picked your birth team well, you can entrust the work of thinking to them. Your job is something else entirely.

What is this frustration, this feeling of being overwhelmed? It is the gathering of the gales before you reach the eye of the storm. If you can believe this, you can get through it.

Instead of seeing the pain as a problem, women who give birth naturally experiment with coping with contractions just as they are. The sensation of each contraction feels like more than you can bear. And yet, on the other side is a truly wonderful feeling of letting go, of finding that you can bear more than you ever dreamed possible, and, ultimately, of making it to the end.

Think of this pain—this contraction—as a mounting ocean wave. Those incoming waves look so intimidating when you are in the water, but if you have faith, hold your breath, and dive into them, you will emerge on the other side. And if going through a wave doesn't appeal to you, how about surfing it? When you are standing on your surfboard on top of those awesome waves, they're not so bad.

When you are facing the challenge of active labor, you must draw on your inner resources to get you through, although your birth team can support and guide you toward those inner resources. Prepare yourself mentally as much as you can by reading about, thinking about, and practicing "letting go."

An example from yoga will illustrate this particular skill. When you move your body into a demanding yoga pose, you can feel pain in your stretching muscles. Holding the position for a minute or longer is an intense physical sensation. While specific muscles contract, the yoga practitioner is supposed to relax all other muscles, breathe slowly and deeply, and consciously let go of tension in her mind and body. When I have done yoga with real concentration, I am always amazed at how differently I experience a yoga pose. This skill—of allowing certain muscles to work without becoming tense elsewhere in your body or anxious in your mind—is what will get you through labor.

For some of us, yoga is the best practice for labor. For others, the best practice is creative work, everyday work at our jobs, or prayer and spiritual activities. Also helpful are childbirth-preparation courses that focus on relaxation. Hypnosis-for-childbirth classes usually teach relaxation skills extremely well. Some Lamaze classes do a good job in this area, too (but many Lamaze classes focus on medicalized hospital birth, so be sure to ask questions before signing up). Practice letting go, trusting, and relaxing wherever this makes sense in your life.

Visualization

Directing your mind toward a positive image—such as an ocean wave, an opening flower, or a rising sun—diverts your attention from pain. This technique has been proven to circumvent unconscious fears, promote the body's production of oxytocin hormones and endorphins, and block unhelpful hormones. Some women are able to use visualization in labor all on their own, but many benefit from being coached. Some visualization scripts are included in the sidebar above. You can use these as an inspiration for creating your own.

Breathing

When I teach childbirth-preparation classes, I do not spend a lot of time on breathing. This is not because breathing is unimportant during birth. Breathing is extremely important. However, most women are able to use breathing to help them cope with labor pain without spending much time practicing in pregnancy.

In labor, you can experiment with how your contractions feel when you hold your breath, when you take shallow breaths, and when you take deep breaths. Most women find that holding their breath during labor increases their sensation of pain. Slow, conscious breathing, in contrast, usually diminishes pain.

If you have a trained doula, she will notice when you hold your breath. When we feel fear, we naturally hold our breath. Some of the key signs that a woman isn't breathing are that her shoulders are tense, her brow is furrowed, and her jaw is clenched. Often, a gentle touch to the shoulders or face is enough to relax those muscles and prompt her to inhale.

Concentrating on breathing is a time-honored method of coping with labor pain. A woman named Laura described to me how paying attention to her breathing changed her experience of labor. Her contractions at 7 centimeters' dilation were so intense that she was on the verge of saying, "I can't do this anymore." Her midwife said to her, "All you can do is breathe."

Those simple words worked for Laura. "I just realized there wasn't anything I could do about this pain. The only thing I had any control over was my breathing. So I stopped thinking about the pain and started thinking about my breathing. And then it suddenly became doable," she said. She stopped concentrating on the pain and devoted her attention to each inhalation and exhalation, trying to make them as long and deep as possible.

Staying Upright and Mobile

Most women find that labor is more manageable when they remain upright and when they are mobile. The worst labor position—psychologically and physiologically—is lying down. If it is just one of many positions you use during labor, lying down may contribute positively to your experience. Generally speaking, however, you are better off *up*. When you're upright, according to one theory, gravity helps your labor. Another theory is that movement stimulates stronger uterine contractions. However they work, these are long-established techniques for managing labor pain, handling a labor plateau (see Chapter Eleven), and stimulating progress.

Your hospital room, however, is designed for you to be a patient in a bed. There is little room for pacing or squatting. You may have to get creative to remain upright and mobile. Many women walk the labor-and-delivery hallways in labor. Some labor in a waiting room, kitchen, or library room on the labor-and-delivery floor. The shower is often a good place to try squatting. Don't be shy about using whatever you need on the labor-and-delivery floor.

Keep moving throughout your labor. As active labor intensifies, you will probably have to remain in one position during the contraction itself. When the sensations subside, however, you can resume walking or swaying or dancing or rocking. Dancing with your partner is a lovely way to spend your time in labor. As a bonus, I have noticed nurses hesitate to pull couples out of an embrace to perform routine tests.

Some time-honored positions to try include:

• walking hospital hallways;

• leaning against the wall or another support;

• sitting on a birth ball on the floor;*

• sitting on a chair, leaning forward, and draping your upper body over a birth ball;

• kneeling backward on a hospital bed, or leaning against a raised back of the bed;

• sitting wide-legged on the toilet;

• kneeling on the floor;

• lying down in a bathtub;

• kneeling or leaning forward on a birth ball in a bathtub;

• resting on hands and knees; and

• sitting on a straight chair backward, leaning against the back of the chair. This position can also be used in a shower.

---

* A birth ball is the sort of large, inflatable ball that is often used at gyms and yoga classes. Ideally, the ball should be large enough for you to sit on with your feet flat on the floor.

Of all these positions, the hands-and-knees position deserves a few words. Some women spontaneously get on their hands and knees and find that this is the most comfortable position for most of active labor and even for delivery. This position relieves the back, shoulders, and legs from the weight of the pregnant belly. It also helps decrease the pressure you might feel from the descending baby pushing on your tailbone. However, it is the position women use least frequently. As a doula, I often remind women that this position is an option. In a hospital, you may have to move some furniture to make space for this position. You can put down a towel or blanket on the floor or use this position in the bed, shower, or tub.

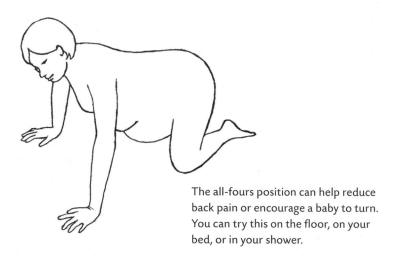

The all-fours position can help reduce back pain or encourage a baby to turn. You can try this on the floor, on your bed, or in your shower.

During your pregnancy, think about at least five positions that you would be willing to try during labor. Practice all five with your labor coach. Think about what props you might need for specific poses. Do you need a birth ball? Extra pillows? A straight-back chair on which you can sit backward? A birth stool?* Plan ahead to make sure you will bring what you need or have it available for your use at the hospital.

---

* Some hospitals and midwifery practices own birth stools. A birth stool looks like a wooden or metal step stool with a top shaped like a half-moon. Sitting on a birth stool is especially helpful if your ankles or legs cannot support you in a squat.

Using Water

In a mother-baby group that I have led for many years, women share their birth stories. Very often they relate the experience of labor in crisp storytelling language until they come to the part when they used water. Then their tone and demeanor soften dramatically as they say something like, "Then I got into the tub. And it was heavenly!"

Not all women experience such dramatic relief from hydrotherapy, but enough do that it should be on your list of options. Generally speaking, if you already know that you relax well in a shower or bathtub, you are an excellent candidate for using water during labor.

Many hospitals have special birth tubs that are large enough for trying out a variety of positions or accommodating two people. But often only one or two tubs serve a whole labor-and-delivery floor. The policy is usually "first come, first served." (Note that few hospitals allow women to give birth in the tubs.)

Luckily, virtually every hospital room has a shower. You might sit on a chair in the shower and direct the water to your belly or sit backward on the chair so the water massages your back. Don't forget that you can get on all fours in the shower, if that feels good. I encourage partners to bring at least two bathing suits and a change of clothes because the partner may decide to get in and out of the water several times.

Even if your hospital does not have a birth tub or showers for labor, or if you have access to a shower but the water pressure bothers you too much during contractions, you can still harness some of the calming power of water. Ask your nurses for two large containers so you can stand or sit with your feet in warm water. A few drops of lavender oil in a footbath can help you stay calm and centered. Or, with warm washcloths, your support person can wash you all over: back, shoulders, face, legs, arms. If a summer labor is heating you up, you might labor in the bathroom with a steady stream of cold water coming from the sink faucet. Between contractions, you can dip your hands into the water or splash your face.

Handling Back Labor

Having back labor means that in addition to feeling contractions in your abdomen, you also feel pain in your lower back. This is, unfortunately, a relatively common experience. Perhaps as many as one in four laboring women experiences some back labor. Often, the cause of the back pain is the baby's position. If the back of the baby's head is against the mother's spine (in a "posterior" position), the heaviest, least flexible part of the baby presses on the mother's back during contractions. This pain can remain even between contractions. Though the posterior position is most often considered the culprit, some women with well-positioned "anterior" babies experience back labor, too.

In late pregnancy, you can stimulate the baby to get into an anterior position by doing "pelvic rocks." Mickey Sperlich, a midwife with more than twenty years of experience, recommends doing one hundred pelvic rocks per day: fifty in the morning and fifty in the evening. By using gravity in this way, you may be able to feel your baby shift toward the front of your belly.

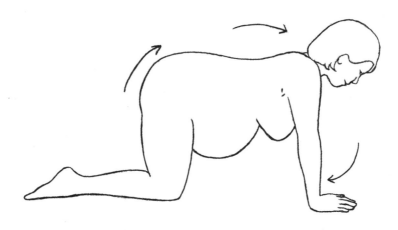

Move your body slowly and with your breath—up and in, down and out—through this pelvic rock.

How to Do Pelvic Rocks

Kneel on the floor with your hands and knees hip-width apart. Without arching your back or exaggerating the movement of your head and neck, tilt your buttocks up toward the sky. The small of your back will naturally curve inward, but you should not exaggerate this effect. Let your buttocks relax downward so that your back is straight and level. Repeat.

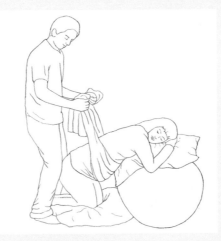

How to Use a Rebozo

Rebozos come to us from Mexico. A rebozo is a long piece of woven cloth that is usually four to six feet (1 to 2 m) long. It is a piece of clothing that Mexican midwives have traditionally used to help women in pregnancy and labor. In labor, a doula or partner can "sift" the birthing woman's belly. This can feel good because it provides a kind of physical support to the woman's belly. It's also useful for encouraging a baby to move position. You may want to try this if labor appears to have plateaued (which could be because of baby's position) or if you know that the baby is posterior. Describing sifting in words is cumbersome, but learning from a demonstration is very easy:

- A great video by Katherine Parker Bryden about how to use a rebozo—and how to improvise one from a hospital bed sheet—is located here: www.youtube.com/watch?v=1p2cd2P63Q4

- Another wonderful resource about rebozos is at: genakirby.com

How to Use Hip Squeezing

Stand upright or lean against the bed or something else for support. Have your support person stand behind you and push inward, with the heels of the hands, at the top of your hips during a contraction. If the pressure is in the right place, you will probably feel relief. The correct position, however, may not be self-evident to either of you, so you may need help. Most doulas and labor-and-delivery nurses are well trained in this technique.

How to Use Counterpressure

Lean against the wall or the bed and have your support person push two fists into the small of your back. You may need to experiment together to find the best placement for optimum pain relief. It may be easier for your support person to push tennis balls rather than fists against your back, as in the illustration. Easiest of all, your supporter can hold the handles of a rolling pin positioned across your lower back. During a contraction, you will probably want constant, firm pressure. As the contraction ebbs, you might enjoy a gentle up-and-down roll of the rolling pin.

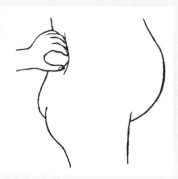

Many women find relief from contraction pain through pressure on their lower back. Using a tennis ball or rolling pin saves your labor companion's wrists.

Moving, laboring on hands and knees, giving attention to your breath, and laboring in water may help you cope with back labor. In addition, you may especially benefit from counterpressure applied to your lower back or hip squeezing during contractions. If either of these techniques helps you, you are likely to want the action for every contraction until the pushing stage. One of the first births I attended when I was an apprentice in a Russian birth hospital was with a woman who had severe back labor. I was accompanied by two other American apprentices. For ten hours, we took turns squeezing this woman's hips during every contraction. At the end of the day, my arms and hands felt like jelly.

Counterpressure on your lower back can be applied with fists, tennis balls, or a rolling pin. Some women appreciate a jet spray from a whirlpool tub directed to the right area. You can even apply counterpressure with your own fists if your support person needs a break.

Resources for Labor

The Birth Partner: A Complete Guide to Childbirth for Dads, Doulas, and All Other Labor Companions, 4th edition, by Penny Simkin

Active Birth: The New Approach to Giving Birth Naturally, revised edition, by Janet Balaskas

Easing Labor Pain: The Complete Guide to a More Comfortable and Rewarding Birth, revised edition, by Adrienne B. Lieberman

Keeping Your Strength Up

Make sure that you pack plenty of snacks and drinks for labor. Digestion slows during labor, and you will probably be so focused on your contractions that you will not feel hungry, but this doesn't mean you should forgo eating. Keeping your strength up is very important. Without a good store of energy, you cannot expect to make it through a demanding labor without getting exhausted.

Snack Tip

A great snack for laboring women is a honey stick. Your coach can cut off the end, and you can suck out the honey between contractions. Honey sticks pack easily and keep well, so get a handful whenever it's convenient during pregnancy and stuff them into your labor bag.

You are probably going to take only small sips and bites, so the easier the food or drink is to consume, the better. Your support team can offer it to you in manageable bits between contractions. Typically, you might manage to eat a bite of banana after each of three consecutive contractions. This may not sound like much, but those three bites might mean the difference between exhaustion and stamina. Good snack choices include honey sticks, miso soup in a Thermos, yogurt (especially the drinkable kind packaged for children, so you don't have to maneuver a spoon), and soft fruit that doesn't require much chewing, such as a banana. I have found that the squeezy packages of fruit and vegetable purees sold in the baby food aisles of most grocery stores are perfect for laboring women. These did not exist a decade ago, but they are now my go-to food for labor. No chewing is required, and vitamins, minerals, and calories are delivered quickly.

Crying or Laughing

I often recommend crying or laughing when labor seems to be stalled. You can read more about these tools in Chapter Eleven.

One of the best ways to practice being fully open with your emotions during labor is to be fully open in late pregnancy. Cry, laugh wildly, go crazy. Enjoy the ups and downs of your emotions as fully as you can. Too many of us try to contain the crazy feelings we experience in late pregnancy instead of riding the roller coaster wherever it might go. Yes, it

The Power of "I Love You": A Note for Partners

If you have trouble thinking of what to say at any time in labor, it is always appropriate to say, "I love you." My husband didn't start saying this wonderful sentence until I started pushing in my first labor. He probably said it about ten times altogether. Every time he said it, I felt a rush of warmth through my body that lightened the pain considerably. In everyday life, I like to hear that he loves me, but the words don't have quite the same magic. In labor, it was like my own private epidural.

Author and natural-birth activist Robbie Davis-Floyd remembers her husband's ability to change her experience in birth, too. She says, "I crouched on the bed in terror and panic and panted to Robert that I could not do it, that I thought I would die. His strong hands grasped my shoulders, and his calm voice said firmly, 'Focus on me.' I peered at him through a fog of agony and fear and his liquid golden brown eyes poured strength, peace, and love into me" (Bernstein, 1993, pp. 190–91).

Before the birth of our second child, I tried to explain to my husband the power of his words. I asked him to say, "I love you" as often as possible. Unfortunately, he didn't completely understand, and I did not spell out exactly what I meant by often. I meant, "Please say, 'I love you' during every contraction." He did say it often, and it had the same warming, pain-relieving effect every time, but he did not say it during every contraction. Later he said, "It felt funny to keep saying the same thing over and over. And it's kind of weird with all these people around to be saying something like that."

By my third labor, I managed to convince him to forget his embarrassment and resign himself to being a broken record. Those little words have such power over my brain and my body. Holding his hand and hearing them over and over in my third labor helped me more than anything else.

may take us through a valley of despair. But it may also take us to heights of exquisite delight. This is the time when you are probably most aware of and moved by the miracle of life. If you allow yourself, you will experience the full glory of the feelings that poets have tried to capture in words for thousands of years. Instead of being a superwoman who remains pleasantly sensible and rational up until the very end, experiment with indulging yourself in late pregnancy.

Using Words of Encouragement

For many people, giving reassurance is not a skill that comes naturally. It must be learned and practiced. Your coach should prepare to witness your emotions in all their magnificence. Consider some of the worst things you can imagine a woman saying during labor:

"I think I'm going to die!"

"I hate you!"

"Don't touch me!"

"I can't do this anymore!"

"I'm so tired."

"I don't think I can do it."

"It hurts. It hurts so much."

"Help! Help me!"

Say them out loud.

Ask your partner or other support person to practice listening to these dramatic words before labor, when they will not induce panic. Ask your partner to offer acceptance and encouragement in return. Ideally, your partner will redirect your energy toward the goal of opening up your cervix, pushing, and having a baby. By practicing with you, your partner will give you permission to say whatever you need to during labor without fear. You may not actually use any of the words on this list while you're in labor, but you should be able to trust your partner to respond positively to whatever you do need to say.

Here are some examples:

You: "I can't do this anymore!"

Your partner: "You're doing it, honey. Just focus on this contraction."

You: "I'm so tired."

Your partner: "You're tired. And you can do it. You are doing it."

You: "I think I'm going to die!"

Your partner: "It's really painful. And you're getting close to the end. Your baby is going to be here. Breathe."

You: "I hate you!"

Your partner: "This is harder than you expected. You're doing a great job."

All the techniques described in this chapter are designed to help you surrender to labor and find a feeling of flow. Finding flow in labor is not so different from finding it in everyday life, in creative endeavors, or in a basketball game. If you are experienced at finding ease in one of these other areas, you will have more confidence in overcoming the necessary chaos to attain flow in labor.

If you have ever felt panic while you were writing a long paper for school, while you were perched at the edge of a ski slope looking down the mountain, or while your three-year-old screamed at the top of his lungs for an hour, you know what it feels like to be overwhelmed. The rational mind does not know what to do. But if you find the strength to push through, to forget the near-impossibility of the task at hand and just do it, you know that sometimes you find the answer. And that it's wonderful when you do. You become a bit stronger, a bit surer of yourself. The next time you face the same situation, you have a memory of the joy on the other side.

The pain of labor can be overwhelming. And you can handle it.

CHAPTER 11

ACTIVE LABOR: WHEN PROGRESS SLOWS

I T IS NORMAL FOR LABOR TO PLATEAU.
Although it is normal to progress 1 centimeter per hour, it is also normal to progress faster or more slowly. It is normal to need time to integrate new sensations and new emotions during labor, and during this time progress may appear to stop. We call these integration periods *plateaus*, a term coined by the midwife Elizabeth Davis (2004). Some studies suggest that it is more common to make progress in spurts than to dilate at a steady pace. The mother may feel stuck at some point, but the stop is just temporary. Anyone who has attended many natural births can tell you stories of labor that seemed to get stuck at a certain point, only to take off like a jumbo jet once the woman made it across the plateau. Yet most women's labors are managed in hospitals as if steady, measured progress is the only possibility, as if only a textbook average is normal.

In a midwifery class at the University of Michigan, nurse-midwife and professor Michelle O'Grady explains to her students that a laboring woman's body has many "feedback loops"—complicated hormonal and physical interactions—that naturally cause labor to plateau. With each centimeter of cervical opening, with each new phase of labor, the body must adjust. More or fewer hormones must be produced. Receptors for each and every hormone must be activated, deactivated, or even manufactured from scratch in cells of the uterus and elsewhere in the body.

O'Grady suggests that we respect plateaus as natural occurrences that give the uterus a break before it advances to the next phase of labor. She recommends that if we decide to intervene, we consider first and foremost whether the woman needs to eat or drink. If she is low on water or energy, her body may be unable to produce enough oxytocin (or other hormones) or receptors to utilize the oxytocin.

If you have reached a plateau, treat it first and foremost with water and food. Try to urinate. And then try to ignore it. Do your best to forget how many centimeters your cervix has dilated.

A plateau can cause you to despair. You can't help but think that you are going nowhere, that all the pain you are experiencing is accomplishing nothing, and that you have far too many hours of this pain ahead of you. If you have been laboring at 7 centimeters for three hours, you think, "How in the world can I make it to 8 centimeters, and 9, and 10?" The calculator in the dark recesses of your brain computes that at three hours per centimeter you have nine hours to go. In fact, you may have only one.

The best approach is to focus on the here and now. Focus on this contraction, not the next one or the one after that or, God forbid, on the one coming in the next hour. (In this situation you will likely need a lot of support. See "A Guide for Your Partner" on page 201.)

Everyone else at the birth desperately wants to see progress, too, so the atmosphere becomes one of fearful watching and constant monitoring. The medical staff do more and more fetal heart monitoring, and the vaginal exams come closer and closer together. The nurses keep poking their heads in to "see if anything has changed." If no one brought up this question, you and your partner might just keep going without feeling discouraged at all.

Try to remember that doing cervical exams (or intervening medically) may be all that the staff know to do. They are probably not used to giving hands-on labor support to women who labor naturally. All they can do is check your cervix, over and over again. They do this because they want to give you the good news that you are progressing. Think how happy it makes a nurse to announce, "Congratulations! You're fully dilated. You can push now. Your baby is almost here."

Remember that a plateau is not a crisis. It does not require any hurried decisions. This is the perfect situation in which to use the vital sentence introduced in Chapter Nine: "We'd like to wait an hour." Putting off cervical examinations helps a lot. In my experience, nurses generally assume that a woman wants frequent cervical exams. They assume that she wants to know if or when she has made progress. When she says, "We'd like to wait an hour" to the suggestion to do an exam, nurses are often willing to back off. They can see the difference between a woman who is determined to make it on her own power and a woman who is looking to them for help and information about her status. That simple statement, respectfully delivered, changes the entire dynamic of the "watched-pot" scenario.

Staying focused on your labor and ignoring the constant monitoring and buzzing about how you are "stuck" may be enough to get you across the plateau. You emerge on the other side, and labor goes on. In some cases, however, the plateau becomes the enemy—something you feel pressed to conquer. You might even be given a deadline: "If you don't get to 7 centimeters by 4 o'clock, we're going to have to do something." Usually, that something is giving you Pitocin, a drug that makes contractions stronger (and presumably, though not necessarily, more effective). When 4 o'clock rolls around, though, you can again say you'd like to give your body the chance to labor naturally and put off Pitocin for another hour. And you can say that again at 5 o'clock and 6 o'clock, if necessary.

Yet, when you've been given a deadline, disregarding the plateau may become impossible after a few hours. In the following sections are some suggestions for handling plateaus that cannot be ignored.

Eat, Cry, and Move

Plateaus can be caused by a number of things. Because you probably won't know at the time what is causing yours, you will need to try a variety of solutions. Time after time, as a doula, I have worked through my bag of tricks, struggling to maintain confidence as each has seemed to fail, only to finally hit upon the action or the phrase that acts as a tripwire. All of a sudden everything starts going gangbusters. Later, witnesses say, "Nothing was happening until you tried X. That really did the trick."

In general, it's best to work through the possible physical causes of a plateau and then move to possible emotional causes. If the related measures don't work, look at baby causes. See the table of possible causes and solutions on pages 198 to 199.

If you become stuck and can't remember much else from these pages, try to remember "Eat, cry, and move." Each of these steps gets at a different kind of labor block.

Because any combination of factors may be blocking progress, combination approaches usually work best. A honey stick may not get labor going all by itself, but if you try eating a honey stick and then walking the hallway, the combination might strengthen contractions.

Many of us are uncomfortable exploring our emotions, especially as they affect our bodies. We think of our bodies as separate from our minds and emotions. Yet, as I discussed in Chapter Two, our bodies and emotions are absolutely interdependent. In labor, this is especially clear.

When hospital staff recommend augmenting a stalled labor with Pitocin, they are addressing possible causes of the plateau: the woman's body is not producing enough oxytocin, or it is not effectively utilizing the oxytocin it is producing, or both. But the staff want to treat the symptom rather than the cause.

If a woman's body isn't producing enough oxytocin, why isn't it? Probably because she is experiencing, perhaps deeply and unconsciously, the fear that labor provokes in many women. This fear blocks oxytocin production and stimulates adrenaline production. The woman's partner, doula, or labor nurse can play a pivotal role here. Addressing her fears, helping her overcome and express them, and reassuring her that she is loved and supported can be just as effective as a drug in bringing on stronger contractions. Encouraging the woman to cry is often very effective, too.

Of all the measures in the table on pages 198 to 199, the two that I find to work most often are eating and crying. I push fluids throughout

The Plateaus of Labor and Some Solutions

PHYSICAL PLATEAUS
PROBLEM: A lack of some physical ingredient is interfering with the labor process.

PROBLEM	SOLUTION
You need water or food.	Drink or eat.
Your body is taking a break and getting ready for the next phase of labor.	Focus on one contraction at a time. Try a bath or shower.
You need rest.	Relax as fully as you can. Try visualization, a bath or shower, lavender oil, massage.
You need to pee. Holding urine in your bladder interferes with the work of your uterus.	Pee.
You need to change position.	Move around between contractions. Try new positions. Be upright.

EMOTIONAL PLATEAUS
PROBLEM: Fear, anger, or sadness is blocking the production or reception of oxytocin, probably by causing the production of too much adrenaline.

PROBLEM	SOLUTION
You are scared at a deep, primal, unconscious level.	• Cry. Your partner can hold your hands and ask earnestly, "Can you let it out with tears? Can I hold you while you cry?" • Scream, out loud or into a pillow. • Try belly laughs. • Your partner can try the words, "You are safe." • Try to get a feeling of grounding. Your partner can experiment with holding your feet or head. Some women feel better when someone holds her feet and another person holds her head, neck, or cheeks.
You are scared about something specific at the hospital.	• Tell the staff you need thirty minutes of privacy. • Cry, scream, or laugh loudly. • Your companion can try the words, "You are safe" or ask, "Are you feeling frightened right now?" • Your companion can hold you in a soothing, enfolding way.

You are afraid of the coming pain and are unconsciously holding back.	• Cry, scream, or laugh loudly. • Your companion can remind you that the future will take care of itself and help you focus on the here and now. • Breathe slowly and deeply. • Your partner can encourage low vocalizations like the sound "ahh." Opening your jaw will help you open internally.
Unresolved emotional issues are blocking you. They could be from your childhood, or they may concern your pregnancy or your relationship with your partner.	Cry, scream, or laugh loudly.

BABY-CAUSED PLATEAUS
PROBLEM: The baby's head is not helping your cervix open.

PROBLEM	SOLUTION
Your baby's head is not fully and forcefully applied to your cervix. (Your baby may be in a posterior position—that is, facing forward—or her head might be slightly tilted.)	• Change position at least every forty-five minutes. Try standing, resting on all fours, squatting, sitting on the toilet, kneeling, sitting on a chair facing backward, or sitting on an exercise ball. • Walk between contractions. Pretend to climb stairs in an exaggerated way. • Rotate your hips to help the baby rotate to a better position. Have your partner firmly squeeze the tops of your hipbones together to open your pelvis more. • During a vaginal exam, ask your caregiver to feel for the position of the baby's head. A tiny amount of pressure in just the right spot can sometimes move the baby's head into a slightly better position. • Ask your baby out loud to get into a better position.
You have the sense that your baby isn't ready to be born. This may be your own emotional block, yet you feel that it comes from your baby.	Talk to your baby out loud about how wonderful it will be to be here, with you, in your arms, in this world.

labor, and when labor seems to stall, I add honey or switch to diluted juice for an energy boost. I used to save the suggestion of crying for a last-ditch effort to get labor moving when the threat of medical intervention loomed. However, crying works so well and so often that I tend to suggest it much sooner now.

Crying is often the hardest intervention for support people to initiate, yet it is often exactly what a woman needs. Usually, she doesn't know it. And that's the whole point. If she knew what she needed to do, she would simply do it. The nurses probably don't feel close enough to her to be comfortable suggesting tears. Paradoxically, offering Pitocin to a woman who deeply desires a natural birth can have exactly the needed effect of causing crying. After being stuck for hours at a particular point in labor, many women break down in tears of disappointment when the nurse or doctor tells them they must have Pitocin. In these cases, I believe, the crying rather than the Pitocin may be more often responsible for progress.

Crying in Late Pregnancy

Many women find themselves weeping for no reason during pregnancy. In our culture, this weepiness is often ridiculed or discouraged. Yet it is nature's way of preparing our minds and bodies for the full release required during labor and in early parenting.

I am such a believer in the value of crying that I encourage my clients to cry as much as possible in their last weeks of pregnancy. Many women later say that they were feeling high highs and low lows during those weeks already, but being given permission to fully express the lows was helpful. I'm not sure whether crying in pregnancy works by releasing built-up feelings or providing practice in opening up and self-acceptance, but either way, it works. For many women, crying is a faster and safer way to express their deepest fears than using words. Some of these fears may be so deep and unconscious in the human psyche that there are no words for them anyway.

Lucy and her husband, Jackson, came to my house for a prenatal consultation. At first, they stuck to relatively "safe" topics regarding Lucy's pregnancy and their birth plans. After about an hour, however, they opened up emotionally. We talked about Lucy's fears that Jackson would not be there emotionally for her during the birth and related

A Guide for Your Partner

When labor plateaus, keep encouraging the mother. Keep telling her that she's doing great, that she is strong and capable, and that every contraction *is* doing important work. She may tell you that she's tired and disheartened because she's "stuck" at a particular number. Ignore the number! If she sees that you are not concerned about it, she will feel freer. Focus on her strength and capability. Tell her that you are proud of her, that you love her. Help her visualize the baby arriving and being in her arms. Suggest changing positions, walking around, drinking water, or eating a bit. When you can't ignore the plateau any longer, you can try these ideas:

- Offer a glass of water with a bendable straw.
- Offer a bite of food, tea with honey, or another drink with calories.
- Suggest to the mother that she pee. If she resists but hasn't peed for more than two hours, suggest this more strongly.
- Invite her to cry.
- Invite her to scream loudly.
- Invite her to scream softly, or to scream into a pillow.
- Invite her to rest. Ask, "How can you rest more between contractions?"
- Suggest a shower or a bath.
- Suggest laboring in the bathroom with water running.
- Try any new position.
- Encourage a change in the way she has been vocalizing. You could chant a new word during a contraction such as "baby, baby, baby" or "yes, yes, yes," or you could moan in a deep voice. Women often follow suit.
- Try one more walk around the labor-and-delivery hallway.
- Talk to the baby out loud or encourage the mother to do so.
- Hold the mother's feet or head to give her a feeling of grounding.
- Ask the hospital staff for thirty to forty-five minutes of uninterrupted privacy.
- Go back through the list. Something that didn't work before may work now.

Focus on this moment. Don't let yourself worry about "what's going to happen" in the future.

those fears to her experiences growing up with parents who were often unsupportive and uninterested. We all felt an emotional shift. Lucy shed some tears that evening. I encouraged her to cry whenever she could in the weeks before her due date, and she did. When I saw her at the birth, in the first two weeks postpartum, and even months later, she said that hearing my voice made her want to cry. "And I usually don't cry," she told me, laughing at herself.

Labor demands letting go of control. Letting ourselves feel deep and scary emotions—like sadness, anger, and fear—before and during labor helps us let go physically. The hard, deep, emotional work that Lucy did in the last weeks of her pregnancy helped her surrender in her labor. Without emotional obstacles, labor can proceed more smoothly. In Lucy's case, labor went smoothly and quickly, lasting about six hours from start to finish.

Crying in Labor

Dakota, her husband, and her mother picked me up in their car on the way to the hospital. Dakota was clearly in early labor, though she really hoped and believed that she was in active labor. We waited about an hour for Dakota's doctor to arrive. It was early morning, and no one was in the offices yet, so we had the floor completely to ourselves. Dakota labored magnificently and confidently in the hallway. I remember watching her against the wall, blowing air quietly through her mouth, which she held in an *O* shape. She was wearing a miniskirt and a long black poncho that draped fashionably over her belly. Her wide-legged stance and dreamy expression gave her a look of complete confidence and inner peace. This snapshot remains vivid in my memory.

After we got through triage and made our way to her hospital room, the nurse handed Dakota a hospital gown and asked her to change. (This is the usual practice in most hospitals, although many women who give birth naturally insist on wearing their own clothing.) Dakota went into the bathroom and put on the gown. When she returned to the room, her entire demeanor had altered. Her confidence had melted from her face and body. In its place was a look of controlled fear. Dakota sat down on her hospital bed, and the nurse began asking questions. Dakota answered the first several questions and then handled a contraction. After the contraction, she tried to go back to answering questions. Yet I could tell that something was wrong.

I went to her side and sat next to her on the bed, putting my arms around her shoulders. I said, "This feels very real, huh? Here you are. It's really happening. It's scary, isn't it?" She nodded her head yes, and tears started slipping down her cheeks. She sobbed for a few minutes while I held her. The nurse waited quietly and respectfully. Eventually, Dakota regained her composure and said, "I'm sorry. I didn't mean to cry." I assured her that crying was helpful and natural. "Please cry!" I said. "It will really help your labor." The nurse agreed. "That's right, " she said. "Crying is a real release."

Later in labor, when Dakota plateaued at 6 centimeters, I suggested crying again. At first Dakota resisted, shaking her head. About half an hour later, I gently reminded her again that crying was OK. This time she put her arms around me and we hugged while she cried. It was just a few moments and a few tears but a release of pent-up emotions and energy nonetheless.

Both times Dakota regained confidence after shedding tears and being supported in her emotional release. She was more herself and more able to find her way afterward.

I will share one more story here. In one birth I attended, a brave and strong woman named Anjali had survived a four-day induction without pain medication and also without any solid food. On the fourth day, when her baby's heart tones were nonreassuring and her cervical dilation had plateaued at 5 cm for more than 24 hours, she agreed to a cesarean. Before the cesarean, she asked to eat a meal. Ironically, after preventing her from eating for four days out of fear of a cesarean, her doctor readily agreed to this request. She cried about the loss of her dream for a natural, vaginal birth as she ate a hearty meal. She had no sooner finished crying and eating, then she made a surprised face and said, "I feel like I have to poop." Well, nurses and doulas know exactly what that means: a baby is descending in the birth canal! The nurse called for backup. Anjali's baby was born vaginally about twenty minutes later. In this case, I don't know whether crying or eating—or the combination—was the key ingredient. But it seemed clear that one or both of these contributed to getting labor going fast.

What Happens When Women Don't Release Fear in Other Ways

One possibility is that they shake.

For the first several years that I worked as a labor coach and midwife's assistant, I was mystified by this phenomenon of shaking. In medicated labors, we understand that the medicine may cause shaking (especially if it contains adrenaline, as epidurals do). Yet, even in natural births, a good number of women—in my experience, a quarter to a third of women—undergo uncontrollable shaking at some point in labor or in the first hours afterward. In the Russian hospital, we interns asked our mentors about this time and again. The Russian doctors and American midwives gave a variety of answers. Most blamed it on muscle spasms caused by the woman's tensing her muscles for so long during labor. Others blamed a vitamin deficiency or dehydration. And still others just shrugged their shoulders and said, "Some women shiver."

In the United States and Canada, I mostly hear birth professionals blame shifting hormones. Certainly, this seems to be part of the answer. Shaking (as well as nausea and vomiting) does seem to coincide with recognizable shifts in labor intensity. These phenomena seem to come with the sudden rise in hormone levels and then subside as the woman gets used to the new levels.

However, my experiences with shaking in other contexts leads me to believe that fear (and the hormones associated with fear) may also play a role. Some years after working in Russia, I observed a psychotherapy group in which women shared stories about traumatic events from their past. Sometimes, these events were so traumatic and horrifying that just speaking about them caused the women to shake uncontrollably. After they processed the memories in words and tears, and once with nothing more than primal-sounding screams, their bodies would shiver and their teeth would chatter. Blankets couldn't warm them or stop their trembling. Their therapist, Eileen Daly, called this behavior a "fear release."

Fear, like intense physical exertion, releases adrenaline in our bodies, and that surge of adrenaline may be responsible for the shaking. In the vast majority of births that I have attended, shaking has occurred right after the birth of the baby or the placenta. The intensity of pushing may cause an adrenaline rush that in turn causes shaking. However, if you have ever felt yourself trembling in relief after a scary moment, you can understand that sometimes this shaking may also be related to the release of fear. A woman might have been afraid that she would die or that her baby would not make it or that she would not be able to withstand the pain after all. Finally, in the end, everything turns out all right, and she releases those pent-up and unexpressed fears by shaking.

One woman, Tanisha, for whom I was a doula, had been awake for almost twenty-four hours after her waters broke. She experienced mild contractions for about four hours and relatively strong contractions for almost twelve hours. She was feeling exhausted and demoralized when she agreed to her first vaginal exam. Before the examination she decided that if she was more than 5 centimeters dilated she would continue laboring naturally. If she was less than 5 centimeters dilated, she would opt for the epidural. All of us assumed that if she was less than 5 centimeters she would have many, many hours of hard labor ahead.

Her nurse pronounced Tanisha's dilation to be 2 centimeters. Tanisha agreed to an epidural. The moment the anesthesiologist told her that the epidural was in place and she could lean back in bed, her body began to shudder. For the next half hour, Tanisha kept begging for more and more blankets, but nothing could seem to warm her up. And then, the shaking stopped. She gave birth to her baby within ninety minutes of receiving the epidural. (Reading stories like these, I hope, helps you to understand that labor does not always progress linearly, but can "leap" or "jump." These "leaps" are more common than most textbooks or reality shows, or even most childbirth education classes, portray. Indeed, when I asked doulas in an online forum about this, I received dozens of stories about such labor surges.)

On the one hand, Tanisha deeply desired a natural birth. On the other hand, she had often expressed severe doubts about her ability to handle the pain. Her husband did not understand her desire for a natural birth and did not offer verbal or hands-on support in labor. Because the pregnancy had been difficult to achieve and then full of medical interventions for a variety of health problems, Tanisha often referred to her body as "defective."

Tanisha's profound fears about the pain of labor and letting go of control may have interfered with her labor, lengthening it considerably.

Once she received an epidural, she went from 2 centimeters to giving birth in ninety minutes. Since the only change was her sensation of pain, I wonder now whether she could have had a considerably shorter overall labor if she had been able to release her fear of pain in some other way. Yet, as Tanisha says, "That's how it had to go for me."

I accept the paradox inherent in this story. I believe that Tanisha's birth experience was exactly as it should have been. At the same time, there is something to be learned from it. Many of us approach birth as a purely physical challenge. Yet, time after time, birth has shown me that it requires the work of a woman's mind, not just her body. The release of fear is a powerful step on the road of natural birth. It can be both the way and the destination: Releasing fear aids labor. Labor, in its turn, aids in the release of fear.

Think of plateaus as a natural part of the birth process. Your body, which has changed so much in the nine months of pregnancy, is changing extremely rapidly during labor. Like a mountain climber, you might need a place to rest as you gear up for the summit. Sometimes, a plateau has strictly physical causes; your body needs to increase the production of oxytocin or oxytocin receptors, you need to urinate or eat, or the baby's head is a bit tilted. Sometimes, the plateau is caused by emotional blocks, the most common of which is fear. At other times, a combination of physical and emotional causes slows labor.

Whatever happens, there is a reason. By asking the question, "What do my body, my baby, and my heart need right now?" you can refute the interpretation that there is a problem that must be addressed with drugs. Try to give your body and your soul what they need at this moment. With the help of your support people, work through the list of suggestions on pages 198 to 199.

Like a mountain climber, you should rest if you can (resting on a steep mountainside can be just as big a challenge as resting during labor), check your fuel (do you need some calories?), try a new path (do you need a position change?), and release your fears so you can be fully present in the moment. Don't look back. Cry if you need to release tension or fear.

Rest.

Eat.

Cry.

Move.

CHAPTER

12

ACTIVE LABOR: CONCERNS ABOUT YOUR BABY'S HEART RATE

Y OUR BABY'S HEARTBEAT IS THE SINGLE most important window through which to glimpse his health. When the heartbeat is strong and responds quickly to environmental conditions (such as the squeezing of a contraction), we can assume that the baby is doing well. Most hospitals require labor-and-delivery nurses to check the baby's heart rate at specific intervals. Usually, this is accomplished in one to five minutes with either an electronic fetal monitor (which requires that the mother lie down in bed) or with a handheld device (in which case the mother can remain upright and active). A "nonreassuring" heart rate, especially if combined with a fever, a labor plateau, or both, is one of the most common steps on the road to a C-section.

Although most of the time routine heart rate assessments reveal that all is well, it is also quite common for a baby's heartbeat to have unusual, "nonreassuring" patterns. A nonreassuring heartbeat can indicate that a baby may be in distress. Real distress means that the baby cannot handle the stress of labor on its body and should be born quickly, sometimes even as soon as possible. Most of the time, though, it reflects something far less worrisome, such as a compressed umbilical cord. Still, nothing is scarier in labor than hearing your medical caregivers express concern about your baby's heart tones and wonder aloud if your baby is in distress.

Because it is so common for women to experience this complication during labor, all pregnant women should prepare for it. It helps to tuck a reminder into the back of your mind, as you go into labor, that babies' heart rates very often sound nonreassuring and that most babies who have irregular heart tones at some point in labor are born healthy (Chandraharan & Arulkumaran, 2007).

If your baby happens to fall into this category, your job is to continue to labor and to remain calm and relaxed. Figuring out whether your baby's heart rate indicates a crisis is not in your sphere. Worry would only complicate the situation. Focus on what you can do: Surrender to contractions, relax your mind when your uterus relaxes, change positions, eat, and allow your birth companions to interact with the hospital personnel about any next steps. Your birth companions should be prepared to ask for the least invasive interventions if your caregivers want to "get more information."

Your caregivers' job in this situation is to monitor you and the baby to determine whether the heart rate irregularity reflects a real problem (your baby is in distress and needs to be born quickly) or the baby just needs some more time or a position change. Unfortunately, their job gets in the way of your job—to labor without fear. It is hard to remain calm while experts are whispering in the corner about possible fetal distress.

What You Can Do

Surrendering to labor is your healthiest response. If the baby's heart rate is, indeed, indicating distress, interventions may become necessary. But worry and panic would only make everything worse for you and for your baby, by flooding your body with adrenaline and decreasing your production of oxytocin, which keeps labor going.

While your care providers keep an eye out for the worst possible reasons for the baby's nonreassuring heart tones, you can concentrate on the much more common, benign reasons and try to do something about them. Most of the time the baby's heart rate sounds odd because of not-so-serious problems such as these:

- The baby's weight is squeezing the umbilical cord.

- The baby's position makes it hard for the machine to pick up his heart rate.

- The baby is asleep.

- The mother's heart rate, which is usually much lower than the baby's, is mistaken for, or heard in combination with, the baby's. This happens more commonly than you might expect.

- The mother has eaten recently, and this has caused a spike in the baby's heart rate.

These are matters you can address. Remember "Eat, cry, move" from Chapter Eleven? For most of these problems (except a heart rate increase caused by a recent snack), moving and eating are your best options.

Move

Changing positions is your first defense. If the nonreassuring heart rate is being caused by the baby's weight on the umbilical cord, you can solve the problem by getting the baby to move. Many women have discovered that a particular position (such as lying on one's back or side or even standing) causes heart rate problems during labor and that a new pose resolves the issue immediately. An all-fours position usually allows the baby to shift the most of all.

One hospital trained its nurses to use position change as the first line of defense when a baby's heart tones were nonreassuring. Nurses know a wide variety of positions to try, even for women who are on epidurals. Using pillows and the adjustability of the hospital bed, they are able to get women upright and change the tilt of the pelvis, which can allow a baby to shift position. One particularly helpful position uses the back of the bed in the fully upright position. A woman kneels backward on the bed and can drape herself over the back. Then, she puts one leg up to the side so she is balanced on one knee and one foot. After a while, she can turn to the other side and repeat there. This position allows women to rest well in between contractions, gives partners and doulas full access to her back and hips in case she likes massage or hip squeezes, and opens up the pelvis more than just kneeling.

What I noticed at this hospital was how this approach (position change first!) helped everyone in the room remain calm: the nurse, the partner, and the mother-to-be. In other hospitals, a nonreassuring heart rate strip can lead to feelings of anxiety and hand-wringing. But having such a positive, proactive measure to try—such as position change—meant no one had to wonder about how to handle the situation.

Eat

If the baby is asleep, a jolt of calories—from a glass of fruit juice, for example—can probably stimulate movement and a different heart rate pattern.

What Your Birth Companions Can Do

This is a time when having two support people, instead of just one, can mean the difference between a C-section and a natural birth. Why? Because in active labor, especially in late active labor, a woman has little energy or mental capacity to focus on what the nurses and doctors are saying. In this situation, a single support person may need to focus *all* his attention on what the medical caregivers are discussing. This can leave the laboring woman without support exactly when she needs it the most.

If you are planning to have two support people, assign their roles ahead of time. Who is going to interact with the nurses, midwives, and doctors during difficult moments, and who is going to keep supporting you? Then, if an emergency does arise, both of your support people will not abandon you to talk to the medical staff.

Your birth companions should focus first and foremost on supporting you in labor. They can also advocate that your caregivers use the least invasive interventions first. There are two less invasive interventions that they could specifically request:

1. *Using a handheld Doppler.* It's best if your nurses use a Doppler (a handheld ultrasound device to measure the baby's heart rate) throughout your labor. If they have been relying on an external fetal monitor (the kind with two belts that go around your abdomen) and it has shown an irregular heart rate, ask them to switch to a handheld Doppler. First, the handheld monitor

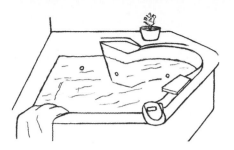

A handheld and waterproof Doppler can give you freedom of movement even in the shower or bath.

allows you to move more freely and try more positions. Second, the Doppler might find the baby's heartbeat in a different place, where it won't be double-counted with your heartbeat or mistaken for yours.

2. *Rubbing the baby's head.* Birth researcher Henci Goer (1995, p. 95) suggests that before a mother agrees to any invasive intervention (such as internal fetal monitoring or a cesarean section), she request that the caregiver try rubbing the baby's head. If the baby's heart rate responds well to the head rubbing, everyone's worries should be allayed. Studies show that checking the baby's well-being by rubbing her head has practically the same level of accuracy as using an internal fetal monitor.

Keeping Your Focus on Your Labor

Most of the time, an odd fetal heart rate by itself is not enough to prompt a medical intervention. Instead, the caregivers watch closely and evaluate all the available physical indicators to determine the best course of action. If your baby's heart rate has been nonreassuring, your caregivers will be vigilant about checking your temperature, your blood pressure, your heart rate, and your cervical dilation. If the baby's heart rate continues to be nonreassuring and one of these other indicators is worrisome, too (for instance, you spike a fever or your labor plateaus for several hours), you are more likely to face pressure to allow serious interventions: breaking the bag of waters, an internal fetal monitor, or a cesarean section.

At this point, maintaining a positive labor is more challenging but also more crucial than ever. Drink water to avoid a dehydration fever. Eat. Change positions. Use all the ideas from Chapter Eleven (pages 198 to 199) to give your body the best chance to progress on its own.

Your primary responsibility is to labor on, even in the midst of a possible crisis. The fact is that I have seen, and so have many other birth professionals, situations like this that are not real crises. In fact, scientific articles about the management of this situation are all about the problem of "false positives." Women give birth vaginally to pink, healthy infants, even after hours of nonreassuring heart tones. They are never explained, but they also never led to a problem. The heart tones were "false positives." I have spent many hours reading articles about how to interpret fetal heart rates during labor. The history of how we have made guidelines and defined problems is fascinating. Suffice it to say, we know less than we wish we did about how babies respond to labor. If you are interested in reading one physician's blog post about how difficult it is to determine a real problem from normal labor, you can find a good one here: www.kevinmd.com/blog/2011/09/doctors-cling-continuous-fetal-heart-monitoring.html.

Concentrating on labor may require great effort on your part, but you can do it. The same techniques that help with the pain of contractions will help you through this situation, too. No one wants to experience complications during labor, but not even a nonreassuring fetal heart rate has to take away your power to labor well.

Laboring well and changing position are the best treatments for a nonreassuring fetal heart rate. There is currently no medicine or procedure to correct this problem in any direct way. By taking deep, calm, measured breaths and visualizing positive images during contractions, however, you can send calming hormones coursing through your blood to your baby. This is something no doctor or nurse can do.

No matter what complication arises during labor, whether it is a labor plateau, overwhelming pain, or a nonreassuring fetal heart rate, you will do best to remain anchored in your body, focused on your labor. The time to think rationally about tests, procedures, and medications is before labor. Any complication in labor can provoke you to feel scared and unsafe. Remember the importance of feeling safe, discussed in Chapter Two? To increase your feeling of safety, take charge of this part of labor that you can control: your focus. By focusing positively on your labor, you may have the power to resolve problems that your medical caregivers can do nothing about.

chapter 13

PUSHING AND GIVING BIRTH

HERE IS THE GOOD NEWS: The pushing stage of labor is usually the part women enjoy the most. The bad news is that a small percentage of women find this "second stage" of labor to be the hardest part.

The reason many women find pushing to be the best part of labor is that they get to put all their might and muscle into the task. Yes, it is hard work, but it is very different from the letting go and surrender of the first stage.

Following are four women's descriptions of pushing. Three of these women describe pushing as easier than labor up to this point, and one finds it harder. In my interviews, three to one was the approximate ratio of those who found pushing easier to those who found it harder.

My favorite part of giving birth is pushing after transition. I think pushing is sensual and exhilarating, not to mention you are about to meet your baby. All the hard work is done, and your body naturally knows what to do. You don't have to think; you just follow. Usually at transition you have met with your last fears or the feeling that "I can't do it"; then come the lovely adrenaline and flow of hormones that make you feel like the most powerful woman on Earth, and you birth your baby.

—Ayesha, mother of three

I remember being in the shower with the detachable shower head spraying hot water right on my back, and then I suddenly had to poop. Then I knew it was transition. I tried multiple positions: hands and knees, on my back, on my side with a leg held up, walking, and squatting, and nothing felt right. I had a feeling of annoyance, but also a feeling of renewed energy, because I knew that the birth would be close, and I felt that I was at a more productive stage of labor. Instead of passively awaiting the next contraction and breathing through it, I now got to do something. I pushed and pushed and pushed, and fortunately labor feels no time, because I pushed for four and a half hours.

—Violetta, describing her first baby's birth

At one point I wondered silently to myself if I could really handle the intensity of the contractions. Then I thought about my grandmother in Florida whose strength I admired and who was nearing the end of her life. I held out, and moments later I was fully dilated. Then there was a pause in the action before the pushing stage, which allowed me to catch my breath. Our doctor asked me if I wanted him to "take the pain away" for the pushing stage. I said no, because I wanted to feel the burning sensation I had read about. Turns out the burning sensation motivated me to keep on pushing. I pushed for thirty minutes. Toward the end, I heard our doctor tell Keith how to put on his special latex gloves and position himself to perform the forearm catch. Together they guided Evelyn's head and shoulders out, and with one final push, out she popped into her father's arms!

During those few minutes right after birth, I felt absolutely no pain anywhere. It was bliss. I remember feeling so relieved at that moment. I sat up smiling and said, "Wow, this is amazing." I had pushed about twenty times, pretty vigorously. I wished someone had reminded me to slow down so that I would not have had to tear. It was a spiritually transformational experience for all of us, and we look forward to bringing other children into the world in a similar way.

—Allison, describing her first baby's birth

Everyone told me that pushing was easier. No one ever said it might be harder. It was way harder. I couldn't believe how much pushing hurt!

—Jaime, mother of one

Positions for Pushing

Position is probably the most crucial element in an easier second stage, yet it is one of the elements over which birthing women have the least control in hospitals. This is because of three factors: the setup of hospital rooms, caregivers' lack of training and experience with various birthing positions, and the psychological state of most women in the pushing stage.

If you were to have complete freedom, you would most likely choose an upright position for giving birth. Most women throughout time have squatted, knelt, pulled on a rope from a ceiling, leaned against a helper, or gotten on all fours to birth their babies. I have rarely seen a woman who has complete freedom decide to lie down to push her baby out. The exceptions are women whose babies are coming exceedingly fast; they may lie down, often on their sides, to slow the birth.

The squatting position is wonderful for the pushing stage. Squatting opens your pelvic bones more than any other position. Since most of us did not grow up squatting in daily life, we are often physically unprepared to squat for long periods in labor. However, if you hold on to something, squatting becomes significantly easier. To visualize how squatting makes it easier to birth your baby, I recommend watching the short, classic video, *Birth in the Squatting Position*. Many childbirth educators own this video and show it in classes, but I also found it on YouTube. The video was made in Brazil in 1973, but is still the best video that depicts this birthing position.

Many hospitals have squat bars, but your partner or doula should be prepared to request one when you start pushing. They are not automatically offered to laboring women. I recommend that you conduct an online search for some images of women using a squat bar in a hospital. You will see many different ways it can be used. One of my favorite methods is to wrap a towel, rebozo, hospital robe, or sheet around the bar for the woman to hold onto.

A supported squat may also be an option. To get into a supported squat, have your coach sit comfortably in a chair. Lower yourself into a squat, facing away, and drape your arms over your coach's thighs. I find that, generally, midwives are more comfortable with catching a baby in this position (which may require them to get onto the floor and set up a sterile field there) than are obstetricians. But I did witness one obstetrician catch a baby when the mother was in a supported squat in the bathroom. It was clear to all of us that she did not have time to move into the main room and climb up on a bed. Her husband sat on the toilet and supported her squat.

As I mention during the birth planning chapters, I highly recommend watching this short but poignant video to give yourself a positive vision of how pushing can be. This video has many wonderful characteristics: a patient care provider who sits below the woman to catch her baby, a supportive partner, loving moments of connection between the mother and partner, use of a rebozo, and an upright position. It can be found at: motherwit.ca/rebozo-assisted-birth and www.facebook.com/pg/humnbirth/videos/?ref=page_internal.

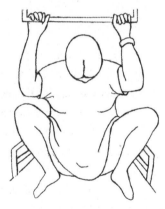

Your hospital room may have a grab bar over the bed, so you can stabilize yourself while squatting.

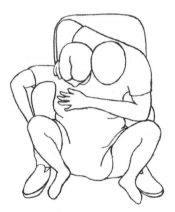

A supported squat allows you to work together with your labor companion during contractions.

Various authors have traced the history of the reclining position, (also called supine or lithotomy position), and its twin sister, the semi-reclining position, to the advent of hospital birthing and doctors as attendants. From the mother's point of view, lying down is not an improvement. It means that the mother and baby have to work against gravity, that the mother loses crucial muscle power for bearing down, and that her pelvis is less open. From the medical caregiver's point of view, however, giving birth in a bed has a lot going for it. The caregiver does not have to crouch down and contort his body for a good view. Instruments can remain sterile on a tray. Birth in a hospital bed is at eye and hand level.

Authors of a Cochrane Review study about women's positions during the pushing stage of unmedicated births wrote this about the supine position:

> *Giving birth in the supine position may have been adopted to make it more convenient for midwives and obstetricians to assist the labor and birth. However, many women report that giving birth on their backs feels painful, uncomfortable and difficult. It is suggested that women in upright positions give birth more easily because the pelvis is able to expand as the baby moves down; gravity may also be helpful and the baby may benefit because the weight of the uterus will not be pressing down on the mother's major blood vessels which supply oxygen and nutrition to the baby (Gupta et al., 2017, p. 2).*

If you have the liberty to move as you wish, you will probably surprise yourself in this stage of labor. Most of the women I interviewed said that the way they had imagined pushing out their first babies was not at all how they actually did it. For instance, some women who desired a water birth found themselves getting out of the water when they needed to push. And women who had imagined giving birth while reclining in the hospital bed found themselves squatting in the shower or on top of the bed.

Most women get an overwhelming feeling that a particular position is the right one. Others benefit from encouragement to try different positions until they find one that feels right. Make sure ahead of time that you and your team are on the same page about what you expect during this stage.

Obstacles to Finding Your Own Position

An unfortunate truth about most hospital rooms (and even many birthing-center rooms) is that the bed takes up most of the space. With a large bed taking center stage, women find it hard to avoid climbing onto it—especially at the end of labor, when a team of medical specialists may crowd into the room. The room is designed for the birthing woman to lie down and for the birthing team to gather around the foot of the bed. As obstetrician Frank Anderson points out, hospital architects do not consider the woman who would like to stand or kneel or squat to give birth. In her case the bed is in everyone's way, and there's no good place for nurses to stand.

Even if your caregiver wants to support you in finding your natural position in which to give birth, she is unlikely to have much experience with positions besides lying down, semi-reclining, and possibly squatting at the end of the bed (if your hospital happens to have beds with squat bars). Because caregivers are trained to attend births in beds, they are most comfortable attending births in beds. All-fours, a position that a substantial number of women prefer for birth, is especially bewildering to someone who has never attended such a birth.

Your caregiver may unconsciously favor a reclining position partially because it is much easier—and more visually rewarding—to check on the progress of dilation and a baby's descent when the mother is lying in bed. As birth becomes imminent, your nurses and midwife or doctor will want to check on the baby with increasing frequency. As a participant at many births, I can tell you it's a thrill to watch a baby slipping down a birth canal. At first, we see just the perineal area bulging. Then, the vagina slowly opens to reveal a sliver of hair and head. When the contraction fades, the head disappears. But as pushing continues, we see more and more head, and the head recedes less and less between contractions. It's amazing to witness.

Your caregivers will miss all this if you give birth in another position. They may not even realize that this is why they suggest you get up on the bed as birth becomes imminent. It takes a lot of trust in the birth process, plus training and skill, to give up the use of sight and rely on touch.

During the pushing stage, women are highly susceptible to suggestion. I have never heard of any experiments that have measured the brain waves of birthing women, but I would wager that at this stage women experience theta brain waves—the ones you experience when you are "in the zone" in sports. In this state, if your caregiver says, "After the next contraction, let's have you get up on the bed," you are likely to do what you are told. Without any argument, you get into your caregiver's preferred position.

They often want you to get into bed at this point to perform a vaginal exam. At the end of active labor, if a woman says she feels "pressure" or the desire to pass a bowel movement, hospital staff will want to determine whether her cervical dilation has reached 10 cm. Though I generally advise against vaginal exams in labor, this is one exam that makes sense to me. It can be useful to know whether there is a cervical "lip" before a woman starts to push. Waiting for the whole cervix to be out of the way of the baby's head is a good idea. At any rate, most of the time a woman will get into bed and lay down on her back for this exam.

In active labor and pushing, changing position usually makes contractions feel worse for one or two sets of contractions. So women do not want to change positions frequently (or even at all). Having just increased pain by getting into bed for the exam, a woman does not usually want to increase it again by immediately moving into another new position.

Also, if the vaginal exam does reveal that you are at 10 cm, you are now *in* the classic hospital birth position. The midwife or doctor is standing at the foot of the bed, between your legs, with gloves on. Your caregiver is likely to put a little pressure on the bottom of your vaginal canal and say, "Push here." And so, your first few pushes may happen this way, with direction from a caregiver, in a supine position. Given all this, it feels as if your position is a "done deal." It can be a socially awkward move to say, "Actually, I want to change this whole scenario up." And, so, women end up staying in this position through the pushing phase.

Knowing that there are obstacles to finding your own way during pushing, you and your companions can prepare for them. In prenatal visits and especially when you present your birth plan, seek assurance from your caregiver that you will be allowed to find your own birth position. Designate your doula or your partner to be your advocate on this matter at the birth. If a nurse, midwife, or doctor asks you to get onto the bed, your advocate can ask you, "Would you like to stay in this position?" All you will have to do is nod your assent.

Pushing Your Way

Women know instinctively how and when to push their babies out.

At the beginning of the second stage, many women do not have a strong urge to push. A good number of women find, in fact, that they have no urge to push. They may be inclined to rest and perhaps even to sleep a bit between the first and second stages. Scientific studies have shown that when a woman waits for the urge to push, her pushes are more effective, she is less exhausted at the end, her baby receives more oxygen (because she is not holding her breath), and she is less likely to tear (Simpson & James, 2005). When you wait for your own urge to push and do not push on purpose just because you've reached 10 cm, it's called "Laboring Down." This was once a rare approach, but it is becoming more and more common, especially at progressive hospitals with midwifery practices.

The great news is that after the first edition of this book, the American College of Obstetricians and Gynecologists came out with guidelines that support a more relaxed, less directed approach to pushing. In 2017, they wrote:

> Collectively, these data suggest that in the absence of an indication for expeditious delivery, women…may be offered a period of rest of 1–2 hours (unless the woman has an urge to bear down sooner) at the onset of the second stage of labor…For most women, no one position needs to be mandated nor proscribed.

Despite this new practice in some places, as soon as your dilation reaches the magic number 10, you will likely be encouraged to push. The most common sort of pushing in hospitals is called "directed pushing." If you watch TV reality shows about birth, you know that often a nurse directs a birthing woman to hold her breath while the nurse slowly (and loudly) counts to ten. Then, the woman is allowed to exhale. Yet many experts believe that it is better for a mother to keep breathing as she pushes for her own and her baby's oxygen levels. If you have read this far in this book, you will not be surprised that my advice on pushing is: do what feels natural to you.

As with position, you will need a strong advocate to help you assert your right to push when and how you want. You cannot push your baby out and tell the nurse, "Thank you for your help, but I'm just going to breathe during these contractions." Someone else must fill this speaking role. For instance, if you're resting when the nurse wants you to push, your advocate can ask you, "You're not quite ready yet, are you?" and you can shake your head.

Your caregiver will want to know throughout the pushing stage that your baby is all right. Your baby's head is designed to change shape and conform to your unique passageway. As the baby's chest descends, liquid is squeezed from his lungs; this is nature's way of preparing the baby to breathe. Your practitioner will check the baby's heart rate often to make sure that everything is going well. In the majority of cases, everything goes perfectly.

Occasionally, a baby's heart rate sounds "worrisome" to the practitioner during the second stage. What should you do in this case? Just keep on working with your urges to push. If your baby's heart rate is nonreassuring to the hospital staff, the only cure is for the baby to be born. Anxiety would just make you tense your muscles and slow your body down.

Preparing for the Big Moment

Many women describe feeling shocked when their babies are born. You have anticipated this moment for months, maybe years. But you have just been through many hours of hard work, and your mind and body are still engrossed in the physical sensations of labor. How can this pain and exertion yield . . . a baby? And yet, miraculously, they do.

Women seem equally divided in wanting and not wanting to see and touch the baby as she emerges. Though few of my interviewees claimed that they knew ahead of time what position would feel right for pushing, they all seemed to know ahead of time whether they would want to see or touch the baby's head in the birth canal. If you think you might want to see or touch your baby, make sure to pack a hand mirror and to let your birth team know of your wishes. In the throes of contractions, you are likely to forget, and the moment is fleeting.

If someone can remind you in the last ten minutes of pushing to get ready to meet your child, you will probably be grateful. Yes, you are pushing through the sensation known as the Ring of Fire. Yet it is possible to be mindful that in seconds a tiny human will be in your arms. You can shift your thoughts and feelings away from your body and toward your baby. When your baby's head finally slips out, and then, with another contraction or two, the shoulders and body follow, you are moments away from the bliss that Allison describes at the beginning of this chapter. You can purposely choose the first sounds your newborn will hear. For instance, you might prepare to say, "I love you," or call your baby by name.

This is another moment when it can be helpful to have a doula or another support person at the birth. If your partner wants to catch the baby or watch the baby emerging, your doula can keep her face near yours.

When Pushing Takes a Long Time

The amount of time it takes to push a baby out varies widely. Some women push for a few moments, others for nine or more hours. A baby may need this much time to shape his head to the mother's birth passage in just the right way. His skull bones are designed to shift position to make birth easier, but this is far from an instantaneous process. Likewise, the mother may need plenty of time to relax and stretch internally.

If your baby is handling pushing and contractions well (that is, the baby's heart rate is good, the head is visible or palpable, and the baby's color looks good), you can push for a long time—probably far longer than you think you can—without endangering the baby or exceeding your own limits of endurance. Though a long second stage is exhausting, it is quite common. Drinking something with a few calories throughout this stage can help you keep up your strength. Changing positions may help, too. Listen to your body to find the position that works best for you and your baby.

Many caregivers start to feel uncomfortable when a woman has been pushing for more than two or three hours. They may wonder whether the baby's head will fit through the mother's pelvis, the baby is not well positioned for birth, or the umbilical cord is causing some interference. They may suggest interventions, including a cesarean section, to get the baby out.

If there is a problem, your caregiver has plenty of time to figure it out. After all, progress is slow. There is no rush to make a decision provided that the baby is doing well. Remember that it is the doctor or midwife's job to worry about complications. Your job is to labor.

Avoiding Episiotomy

I've never met a woman who said, "I am really hoping for an episiotomy." Most of us would do just about anything to avoid a scissor cut in the perineum. Episiotomies are medically necessary in very few cases, to accommodate forceps, for instance, or when two more minutes of pushing might make a critical difference for a baby whose heart rate has been slipping. Rarely, a doctor or midwife can see that a woman is likely to have a "fourth-degree" tear—a tear into the rectum—and performs an episiotomy so that the tear goes to the side rather than to the back. Most North American physicians, however, make episiotomy cuts to the back, toward the rectum, not to the side as doctors do in many other countries, so even this justification is often without merit.

Though you may have discussed episiotomy with your caregiver during a prenatal visit, he may not remember what you decided, and you may be attended at the birth by a different midwife or doctor anyway. Again, your partner or your doula must be ready to advocate for you. When you start pushing, your supporters can ask a nurse to prepare hot compresses. Holding a hot compress against a woman's perineum is a time-honored way to help tissues relax and soften so they won't tear and a cut won't be needed.

Hands and knees is a good position for avoiding tears. If you are going to tear with delivery, though, tearing is probably much better for you than being surgically cut. Tears tend to be more superficial and quicker to heal than cuts. And cutting can actually create more tearing than it avoids. Think about a piece of paper: If you pull on both sides, it does not tear easily. But if you make a small nick in the center and then pull on either side, the sheet is likely to split right down the middle.

If episiotomies are rarely required but often executed, what can you do to improve your odds of avoiding one? Many women massage and stretch the vaginal area in the last few months of pregnancy and swear that this helps. You can also research pelvic floor exercises that are good for pregnancy. In the old days, women were told to do many Kegels to prepare for birth; however, that advice ignores the reality that women need not only tight, strong vaginal muscles, but also muscles that can fully relax and stretch. Doing Kegels properly involves fully relaxing the pelvic floor as well as tightening it. Most practitioners now recommend a combination of squats (for flexibility and stretch) and Kegels (for strength, but also for full relaxation of these muscles). More in-depth research is available about pelvic floor health today than ever before. During delivery, you can have your caregiver press on your perineum with a warm compress. But I am convinced that the best prevention is giving birth in your natural birth position. For the prevention of episiotomies, in fact, almost any position is better than lying down or semi-reclining.

Pooping

A chapter on pushing would not be complete without a note on pooping. The idea of defecating in front of other people horrifies us. Yet it happens every day, at births around the world. When the baby's head puts pressure on the rectum, anything in the way comes out. The good news is that all you care about at that instant is getting the baby out. Even if you have agonized over the thought of pooping in labor for all forty weeks of your pregnancy, when the moment arrives, you will not spare it a second thought.

I often tell my clients a funny but graphic story about Sam from California. This story illustrates that our sense of propriety can change dramatically during labor. Before her baby's birth, Sam would crinkle her nose and speak with great aversion about her husband or others witnessing her poop in labor. During her labor, Sam loved being in a big whirlpool tub, and her midwife was comfortable letting her give birth in the water. The midwife warned Sam, however, that if Sam pooped in the water she would have to get out. As she pushed and pushed and birth was imminent, she did indeed poop in the water. Then her midwife changed her mind and said that Sam could stay in the water as long as the poops were solid. The midwife fished out two tiny, hard stools from the water with a net, and Sam kept laboring. Afterward, Sam remembered thinking, "Thank goodness they're hard!" because she couldn't imagine having to climb out of the tub to give birth. Now, she laughs about the experience. Before the birth, she prayed she wouldn't poop at all. During the birth, she prayed for hard stools. As the children's book says, "Everybody poops!"

If you want a final good reason to avoid the lithotomy position, ask yourself if you'd rather poop with all eyes on your bottom or if some other position, like squatting or kneeling, might not be more comfortable.

The Placenta

In the first moments after birth, while you concentrate on discovering your newborn, your caregiver will be thinking about the placenta.

Delivering the placenta is such an afterthought to the whole birth experience that most women do not include it in their birth stories at all. Your caregiver will watch your belly and the umbilical cord and probably suggest when it is time to push out the placenta. Some caregivers or nurses will offer to show you the placenta, if you are interested. If they do not offer and you are interested, make sure that you have appointed someone on your birth team to ask.

For this "third stage" of labor, you should decide ahead of time how you feel about prophylactic Pitocin. Hospitals have almost universally adopted the protocol to administer Pitocin as soon as the baby is born, even if the mother has had no drugs during the birth, to prevent the possibility of postpartum hemorrhage. The Pitocin is either injected or, if the mother already has an intravenous drip, added to the IV solution. Women who have worked hard to achieve a natural birth sometimes want to remain pharmaceutical-free. Your preference can be written in your birth plan, but your birth companion should know how you feel and be ready to advocate for you. This is a good topic to explore with your childbirth education teacher and caregivers so you understand the pros and cons of this practice. If prophylactic Pitocin is standard protocol, you may have little or no warning that it is coming.

Your Baby Is Born

"My first thought after she came out was 'I have to do this again!'" remembers Janice, describing her second baby's birth. She had experienced myriad unwanted interventions in her first labor, including the use of forceps and suction to pull her baby out. In this second birth, planned to ensure that it would be as natural as possible, Janice experienced the best of what the pushing stage has to offer: triumph and euphoria.

In your own time and in your own position, you and your baby will most successfully navigate this dramatic second stage of labor. Pushing your baby out represents the line between being pregnant and being a mother. Being fully conscious of this moment will allow you to experience its full wonder. This is the vista point of your mountain climb, the end of your marathon, the pot of gold at the end of your rainbow. Savor this culmination.

Congratulations! You have a new baby!

CHAPTER 14

AFTER LABOR

W HEN YOUR BABY IS BORN, your natural birth experience is not over! These next hours and days are still deeply connected to the birth. In later months, if all goes well, the birth and these early days will blur together in a fuzzy postpartum memory punctuated by a few poignant, clear moments. Your baby's natural birth should transition smoothly into weeks of breastfeeding, dozing, smiling at your little one, and joyfully, though perhaps tearfully, connecting with the loved ones who come to see your baby.* The worries of daily life should be far away. Your most important job is taking care of yourself and your new little one.

For many first-time mothers, especially those who did not grow up around infants and children, the early postpartum period can be full of fears about "doing it right." You may be changing a diaper, bathing a slippery and tiny body, and feeding a baby for the first time. These postpartum fears are natural; even experienced mothers feel some of them. Fear is an indication that something valuable is at stake. Dana Gramprie, a counselor in Ann Arbor, Michigan, says that "fear is excitement without the breath." Hard as it is to believe, those tingly, alert feelings that we so often associate with anxiety can also be the sensations of excitement.

---

* Because breastfeeding is an extension of natural birth, I assume in this chapter that you plan to breastfeed. There are, of course, rare but good reasons that preclude breastfeeding.

This simple realization can shift your experience from worry to pleasure. So take some deep breaths and revel in these deep feelings.

Relaxing on Purpose: Your Babymoon Begins Your Fourth Trimester

The first hours after my babies were born, I felt physically raw, vulnerable, and open. And I also felt emotionally raw, vulnerable, and open. "It's like you are connected to all mothers everywhere," says Sujatha. Barbara Harper, author of *Gentle Birth Choices* (2005, p. 24), writes, "Within the first few moments of birth the mother's body will experience the high of a lifetime."

A strong cultural pull to return to normal as soon as possible often prevents women from honoring these intense postpartum feelings. Many women tell "superwoman" stories about their quick returns to work, shopping, exercising, and other activities after delivery. Unfortunately, the natural-birth movement of the 1960s and 1970s encouraged this behavior. In an attempt to make birth seem less like a sickness and more like the healthy activity of a healthy body, natural-birth activists stressed the capability of the female body to get right back to real life after giving birth. Activists convinced women and hospitals that we should go home soon after giving birth (usually within twenty-four hours) instead of staying in the hospital for several days. To the great benefit of insurance companies, this became the new norm.

The unintended side effect, however, was that many women came to think that they shouldn't linger in the postpartum afterglow. They were supposed to master breastfeeding, mothering, and the nighttime care of an infant, make sense of all the well-meaning advice of friends and family, and adapt to a changed relationship with a partner within a few hours or, at the most, a few days. And then they were supposed to be back to their usual routines. If this felt hard, women would often blame themselves and think they were doing something wrong.

In recent years, many midwives have promoted the idea of a "babymoon"—a special time set aside to heal physically and to enjoy the unique weeks after giving birth. Two midwives in California tell their clients they should "cocoon for two weeks and nest for six weeks." But babymoons, cocoons, and nests are all just the beginning of the stage we are increasingly coming to understand is really the "fourth trimester." Babies still need to be treated as a "part of" their mothers in this sensitive period.

Most cultures around the world treat the mother-baby dyad as deserving of rest and special care for the first few months of a baby's life, and most countries support moms and babies financially in this crucial period. I know from personal experience that Canadian parental leave policies make it much easier to relax in the first weeks and months than do U.S. policies. Babies have often barely adjusted to Earth's night-day rhythms at the end of three months. New mothers are still struggling to get out of the house with a packed diaper bag, a fed and freshly-diapered baby, and their own hair combed by the time most U.S. employers demand that they return to work. In my book, *The Fourth Trimester Companion*, I explain much more about how newborn babies have unique sleep patterns and need virtually constant human contact and access to breastfeeding in the first three months of their life.

Advocates of babymoons recommend that during the early cocoon phase, the new family should accept offers of meals and gifts, but they should not socialize. The partner should ideally stay at home with the mother and baby for at least two weeks. If the partner must return to work during this period, or if there are older children in the household, the couple might think about inviting a relative or friend into the cocoon or hiring a postpartum doula. (For many women, having a friend or relative stay in the home is a wonderful choice; for others, it is a disaster. Think carefully and make sure that anyone who is allowed into this treasured time and space will enrich your experience, not drain you.)

Bridget Lynch of Community Midwives in Ontario and past president of the International Confederation of Midwives has researched the postpartum period in-depth. She advises women that the special feelings of this time are fleeting and precious. Instead of trying to "get back to normal" as soon as possible, she recommends protecting and honoring this extraordinary time. Participating in ordinary life too early stimulates the rational, thinking side of our brains. This stimulation can cause us to lose access to the parts of ourselves that have been opened up by birth. Lynch recommends staying in pajamas for two weeks after birth and avoiding touching money or credit cards for the same period. Dressing in pajamas signals that you are in a dreamy, otherworldly state, not quite ready to participate in daily chores or conversation. For comfort in these early days, you might buy new pajamas or a nightgown that opens easily in the front or a bathrobe that zips rather than ties.

The First Hour

A babymoon begins immediately after birth. Most babies, especially those free from the effects of narcotics, are quite alert for the first hour or two after birth. Their eyes are wide open. They look around and gaze into people's eyes. They actively root for the mother's breast and open their mouths with quiet insistence. If they are left alone, unswaddled, they startle themselves over and over again by the movement of their own arms and legs. If they are warmed in someone's arms, they are usually contentedly attentive to the world.

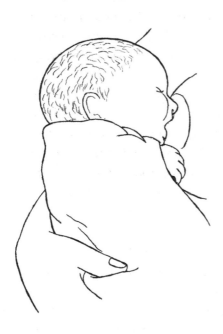

An inspiring video called *Delivery Self Attachment*, by the physician Lennart Righard (1992), is screened in many natural-childbirth classes. It shows newborns crawling up their mother's bellies, bobbing their heads to find their mother's nipples, and latching themselves on to breastfeed without help, all within minutes of being born. Though this does not happen at most births simply because we usually want to hold our newborns in our arms and touch them with our hands right away, the video reminds us that babies are designed to thrive even from the first moments of their life.

This first hour is the ideal time to begin breastfeeding, even if your placenta has not yet emerged. Beginning breastfeeding may not mean that you achieve a perfect latch right away. Giving your newborn time to smell, move around, and lick your nipples is important, too. Many new mothers breastfeed through delivering the placenta, perineal stitching (when necessary), and afterpains. While the delivery of the placenta is usually painless, stitching may be uncomfortable. Afterpains, painful contractions of the uterus as it returns to its prepregnancy size in the early postpartum hours and days, are common in mothers who have birthed more than one child. Although the discomfort of stitches or afterpains occasionally precludes a mother's holding and bonding with her baby, most women appreciate the distraction their newborns provide.

If you're a first-time mother, you will probably appreciate some help from a nurse, doula, friend, or relative in arranging the pillows, the baby's body, and your own arms in a comfortable position. Although many babies are ready to suck right away, some are more interested in smelling, licking, tasting, and just being close to the mother's breast. By licking you, the baby starts to ingest bacteria that are beneficial for her intestines (World Health Organization, 2010). Your helper can show you how to stimulate the baby to open wide and then pull her onto the breast at the right time. Remember, though, that your baby's first experience at the breast should be pleasant, not goal-oriented. Enjoy watching and holding your newborn as you begin this new stage of your relationship.

In progressive hospitals, nurses, doctors, and midwives routinely clean and examine newborns right in their mothers' arms. Since the first edition of this book, more doulas across the United States and Canada report that this skin-to-skin period has become standard practice in their communities. While you hold your baby, a nurse can quickly rub her down to clean off any blood or fluid and scan her for any obvious problems, such as an open spine or breathing difficulties. There will be plenty of time later to weigh and measure the baby and perform routine tests.

In less progressive hospitals, many procedures that can be safely delayed are instead performed immediately after birth. Just because it is the staff's routine doesn't mean you have to acquiesce. Many mothers ask to delay these measures because they can interfere with the enjoyment of the precious moments when a brand-new baby is alert and interactive. Some of the most common practices that can be deferred are injecting vitamin K, sticking the baby's heel for blood samples, and dropping antibiotic medication in the baby's eyes. This is another opportunity to exercise the helpful sentence "We'd like to wait an hour." The eye ointment, which blurs a baby's vision, is better given when the baby gets sleepy and is no longer gazing around. If your hospital administers a first set of vaccines at the time of birth, you can decide to delay these for days, weeks, or even months.

To maximize bonding time, I recommend that you delay any tests and procedures that are not necessary to keep your baby alive. You can easily insert a sentence in your birth plan to this effect: "We would like to delay all procedures or tests such as vitamin K, eye ointment, and the heel prick until the baby is more than an hour old." Your support person should be ready to intervene in the likely case that the hospital staff have not read your birth plan.

Some natural-leaning parents decide to forgo some or all these tests, vaccines, and other procedures altogether. Making informed decisions about medical treatment of your newborn is one of your first jobs as a parent. If you would like more information on this subject, please refer to "Reeferences," pages 263 to 267, for some suggestions on how to begin your research. You may conclude that some of these procedures are more benign than others. You will find that some are required by law, though state laws vary. In many instances, parents can legally refuse medical procedures that they deem unnecessary or potentially harmful.

When Bonding Must Be Postponed

Probably you have written in your birth plan that you would like to hold your baby immediately after birth and stay with your infant all the time that you are in the hospital. Sometimes, because of a problem with either the mother or the baby, the two are separated after birth. The separation may be short, perhaps just a few minutes in the delivery room. And sometimes the separation lasts much longer—hours, days, or even weeks—while the baby is cared for in the neonatal intensive care unit (NICU).

Common Medical Interventions at Birth

Vitamin K shot: Vitamin K is given to prevent a rare but serious bleeding disorder in newborns. Though most mothers who give birth naturally agree to this injection, some prefer to use other preventive methods. For more information see information about the injection at: evidencebasedbirth.com/evidence-for-the-vitamin-k-shot-in-newborns/. If you do decide to forgo the injection or use an alternative treatment, be prepared for significant resistance at the hospital.

Eye ointment: Antibiotic eye ointment can prevent blindness in babies who are exposed to certain bacteria in the birth canal. If you do not have a sexually transmitted disease, your baby does not need the eye ointment. The hospital cannot know for certain whether a mother has such an infection, however, and so the treatment is given to all babies. Also, though this is a sensitive subject, you may not always know whether your monogamous partner is being faithful. If you do decide to forgo it, be prepared for significant resistance.

Heel prick: This procedure allows your baby's blood to be tested for a host of genetic metabolic disorders, usually including sickle-cell anemia, phenylketonuria, and cystic fibrosis. Since a close friend of mine struggled to get her newborn diagnosed with cystic fibrosis, I have a more personal appreciation of this test. It was not included in her state's standard battery of tests at the time, but it is now. Each state tests for its own list of disorders. Many of these diseases are best treated right away (like cystic fibrosis), so medical professionals and most parents find the heel prick useful. It is usually required by law.

Hearing test: Some hospitals perform a hearing test on newborns. Electrodes are taped to the baby's head and headphones inserted in his ears. While sounds come through the headphones, a computer measures the baby's brain activity to determine whether he can hear the sounds.

Vaccinations: The only vaccine that the U.S. Centers for Disease Control and Prevention (CDC) recommends for newborns is for hepatitis B. (Hepatitis B is a serious disease that is spread through sexual contact, intravenous injections, and contact between mucous membranes and infected bodily fluids. If you have hepatitis B, your baby will need treatment and evaluation.) All other vaccines, according to the CDC, should begin no earlier than two months of age. If your hospital administers vaccines other than hepatitis B at birth, you may safely defer.

Separation for the Mother's Health or Recovery

Some women find the immediate postpartum period to be psychologically disorienting or physically challenging. In such a case, plan to let your partner, doula, or a friend or relative hold and care for your newborn while you recover. The airlines remind us every time we take off that in an emergency, it is important to take care of ourselves first so that we can take care of others.

Diane, a mother in New York, remembers that her doula was handing her the baby swaddled in a warm blanket at the same time that the midwife began stitching a tear in her perineum. Though the midwife used anesthesia, the sutures felt surprisingly painful. For about twenty minutes, this new mother could not focus on her newborn at all. Instead, her sister held her hand and talked her through the procedure while the doula held the baby. When the stitches were in place, Diane says that she emerged "from a fog" and "finally noticed that there was a baby in the room." Later, she expressed guilt about not being able to hold her baby during the suturing, but her birth team reassured her that she had made the right choice. Holding the baby while she was in distress would not necessarily have been good for her or the baby.

Carmen, a second-time mother in Ohio, recalls feeling so dizzy from a whirlwind thirty-minute labor and delivery that she needed almost forty minutes to recover. Without the usual hours of labor to prepare psychologically for the birth, she says she felt disoriented and unable to really believe what had happened. Her husband held the baby until she was ready to do so.

Finally, Jessica tells of her experience of losing too much blood after giving birth to her son. Her husband held the baby while the medical team whisked Jessica to an operating room, where she received several transfusions. Her loss of blood left her feeling extremely weak, and she was not able to care for her newborn, even to breastfeed, for several weeks. She did not recover her full strength for many months.

In all these cases, the mother had to rely on others to take care of both her and the baby. These three mothers all went on to bond happily and easily with their babies later.

Separation for the Baby's Health

More and more hospitals are respecting the natural connection between mothers and babies. Nurses are increasingly skilled at carrying out routine procedures while the baby is in the mother's arms. That said, there are still many times that babies are taken away from their mothers for tests, procedures, or therapies—some necessary, and some unnecessary.

If the birth team noticed meconium (the technical name for a baby's first poop) when your bag of waters broke, or if your baby has trouble breathing at first, the medical team may take your baby directly to a newborn bed in your hospital room. Both of these situations are relatively common and, in full-term infants, usually resolve quickly. While lights overhead warm the baby, the team usually suctions the baby's nose and mouth to remove meconium or other obstructions and may give the baby oxygen. From the medical team's perspective, the infant bed is the easiest place to deal with these problems. From the mother's perspective, these may be the scariest and loneliest moments of the birth. Everyone is busy taking care of the baby, and the mother has no idea how serious the problem is. At this point, she may not even know if the baby is a girl or a boy.

Because this scenario is (unfortunately) common, it is helpful to plan ahead for it. Make sure your support people will communicate with you about what they see, so that you do not feel left out and worried. Even in the midst of what looks like a flurry of emergency procedures, your partner or doula can repeatedly ask the staff to do as much of their work as possible with the baby resting on your chest or abdomen. You and your supporters can start talking to the baby right away, calling her by name, even from across the room. I have noticed that when a mother is talking and singing to her baby, the hospital staff seem more aware of her presence and tend to bring the baby back to her more quickly. A newborn is well-attuned to her mother's body and calmed by her voice, her heartbeat, and the smell of her skin (Feldman et al., 2014). If a baby is having trouble adjusting to life outside the womb, it only makes sense that being in the calming presence of her mother should help, rather than hinder, the baby's progress. This is beginning to change at some hospitals, and it seems as though managing meconium births and breathing difficulties with skin-to-skin contact is going to become more standard.

Occasionally, the baby's condition is considered so serious (or potentially serious) that the pediatric staff decide the baby should be admitted to the NICU. The mother may need to deliver the placenta or wait for sutures before she is able to follow the baby to the NICU. In this case, having two support people is extremely helpful. One can go with the baby to the NICU, and the other can stay with the mother. Some families find that seeing pictures on a digital camera helps the new mother feel connected to the newborn in another room.

In mother-baby support groups, I am always astounded at how the moments or hours of separation are remembered with such agony. Women who have just given birth have a deep need to be with their infants. From an evolutionary standpoint, this is only natural. Nature expects that mother and baby will be together, so separation can feel excruciating.

Giving birth naturally is the most reliable path to the elation of holding your newborn in her first moments of life. Yet, even when we do everything possible to ensure a trouble-free delivery, occasionally Mother Nature has other ideas. Though bonding in the first hour is wonderful, humans are fully capable of bonding strongly with their infants hours and days after birth, too.

Jaundice

A special word is called for about jaundice, a common though usually minor problem in newborns. Caused by a buildup of bilirubin in the bloodstream, jaundice produces a yellowing of the skin and the whites of the eyes. It can be a serious problem if it doesn't resolve, but infant jaundice usually resolves easily after a day or two as the baby consumes colostrum (the nutritious liquid that babies receive at the breast before breast milk comes in at about the third day postpartum) and breast milk and then poops out the bilirubin. Treatment in a NICU is not always the best option, especially if it causes separation of mother and baby, thus increasing stress for both and interfering with round-the-clock breastfeeding.

If there is concern about jaundice in your newborn, ideally your baby's doctor will encourage you to breastfeed and to expose your baby's skin to sunlight. Even through a hospital window in the winter, sunlight can help correct jaundice. In the NICU, special "bili lights" are used instead. You should be able to rent such lights for use at home. Studies of home photo-therapy suggest that it is not only good for the family but cost-effective for hospitals and insurance companies (Walls et al., 2004). If your baby is being monitored for jaundice, be sure to explore your options before you agree to several days in the NICU.

The First Three Days

About one to two hours postpartum, most newborns get very sleepy, and new mothers usually find themselves ravenous. After a good meal, the new mother often benefits from a long sleep herself. Parents who are expecting sleep deprivation from the very beginning are often pleasantly surprised to find that their infants sleep almost all the time in the first three days (these parents are less pleasantly surprised when the sleepiness wears off). Many, though not all, newborns sleep so deeply in the first few days that they are difficult to wake up. Though the prevailing wisdom is that newborns should be fed every three to four hours (and awakened if they do not wake themselves to feed), I usually advise new mothers to sleep as long as they can immediately after the birth and an hour or two of bonding. After this first long sleep, you can start waking your baby for feedings if necessary.

The urge to socialize with friends and family may be quite strong because of the excitement of the birth and the intense hormones of the immediate postpartum period, which are designed to help you bond with your baby. The opportunity to sleep will be short-lived, though, so try to discipline yourself to delay the socializing for at least several hours.

The ride home from the hospital can inspire strong feelings in new mothers. You are leaving a safe place, full of supportive people who are experts in caring for you and the baby. The responsibility for this new life feels enormous. You are also taking your infant into a car for the first time. Even if you've prepared for this trip—by installing the car seat in advance, having a specialist check the installation, and then making sure the baby is latched in properly—you may still feel overwhelmed at the thought of the vulnerability of all car passengers. You may also face a momentary dilemma: If your partner or friend is driving the car, should you sit in the front with the adult or in the back with the new baby? Though this moment is fleeting, it represents the first of many such dilemmas that new parents encounter.

These first three days are often hard to remember later but full of wonder and excitement. Plan to enjoy them!

Day Four Postpartum

Around day four after a natural birth, a shift occurs for the newborn and the mother. The baby usually emerges from his sleepiness (though some babies remain quite sleepy for two weeks or so), and his appetite begins to stir. Not coincidentally, around this same time milk starts to fill the new mother's breasts. The emotional high of the birth wanes, often (though not always) leaving in its place a sort of melancholy. As a doula, I schedule a home visit around this fourth postpartum day and usually find women in a temporary funk. They often cry and feel overwhelmed. They are tired and may feel dread about the upcoming night with the new baby.

Usually, they first need to reflect on the birth experience. A woman who has undergone an unplanned C-section or who has had to battle unsupportive hospital staff members understandably has strong feelings to express in the postpartum period. Even a woman whose labor and delivery seemed picture-perfect from the outside usually harbors some regrets. For instance, a woman who experienced a ninety-minute labor might need to complain about the intensity of her labor, though everyone around her says, "You're so lucky!" Another woman might be disappointed that she did not get to give birth in a squatting position or use a birth tub. Voicing these disappointments allows them to fade away and heal.

This is also the time of a shift in the breastfeeding relationship. The experiences of breastfeeding colostrum, in the first few days, and breastfeeding milk can be quite different. Babies and mothers have to learn how to handle the greater volume of breast milk. In many cases, this happens easily and naturally without much outside help. Still, it is an adjustment, and the mother and baby benefit from time alone together. Even well-meaning comments from friends and relatives can interrupt and, unfortunately, sometimes undermine this delicate work.

In cultures with high rates of extended breastfeeding, there are often lactation experts among a woman's family, friends, or neighbors. In North America, however, we often need professional support for breastfeeding. Lactation consultants, La Leche League leaders, and doulas give active help and encouragement to a growing number of women every year. Their advice is based on experience with many lactating women. Professional lactation consultants know much about breastfeeding that even most pediatricians do not. Many hospitals have lactation consultants on staff, and pediatricians should be able to refer their clients to lactation consultants in private practice. You can find a local La Leche League leader online or by calling 800-LALECHE.

Some common challenges in this period include engorgement and concerns about milk flow. Some mothers' breasts are painfully engorged in the first day or two after their milk comes in. Engorgement is best resolved by increased suckling. Unfortunately, it can be difficult or even impossible for some babies to latch on to engorged breasts (in this case, express a little milk to soften your nipples), and some babies are so sleepy that considerable effort is required to wake them. For other mothers, milk flows so fast that the breasts leak all the time, necessitating frequent changes of clothes or nursing pads. Sometimes, the flow is so fast that the baby cannot swallow fast enough and gets irritated.

For still others, this period ushers in weeks of worry that there isn't enough milk to nourish the baby. Although in reality very few women are unable to produce enough milk, this worry is common. Often, the anxiety arises because a baby acts fussier than the parents expected because the woman doesn't feel the tingly sensation of milk letting down or because her milk is slow to let down when she uses a breast pump. As a leader of new mothers' groups, I find this anxiety about "inadequate milk supply" to be widespread. If you have doubts about your milk supply, a breastfeeding counselor can help you evaluate your situation realistically. Most likely, you will discover that you are producing just the right amount of milk for your baby. In the rare case that the baby is not gaining enough weight and is not producing several wet diapers a day, a breastfeeding professional can help you solve the problem yourself or get medical help, if needed.

Friends and relatives who have respected your privacy for several days may unwittingly find themselves visiting a weepy mother and unsettled baby around this time. In this case, their first view of the fledgling breastfeeding relationship may be negative. In a sincere effort to help, friends and relatives may suggest using formula or allowing someone to

Breastfeeding Problems and Solutions

PROBLEM	SOLUTION
Engorgement	Wake the baby as soon as engorgement begins.
	Nurse at least every three hours. Much more frequent feedings are entirely normal.
	Express some milk (into a cloth, in the shower, or into a sink) to soften the nipple area enough so that the baby can latch on and reduce the pain of pressure.
	Use a cold compress or line your bra with a few leaves of cabbage to reduce the pain.
Fast-spraying milk	Let your milk spray onto a cloth or diaper before nursing.
Leaking	Give up clothing! Line your couch and bed with bath towels to absorb leaking. If you're more comfortable wearing a bra, line it with disposable or washable nursing pads.
Sore nipples	A poor latch is the usual cause. If the soreness does not resolve within twenty-four hours, get help to make sure that the situation does not worsen.
Baby won't latch on	You will probably benefit greatly from the help of a lactation consultant.

babysit while you take a break. Such genuine efforts to help will probably feel wrong to you.

You are more likely to need others to quietly and unobtrusively support you by taking care of other business (laundry, dishes, cooking meals, returning phone calls, entertaining other children, and so on) rather than to babysit the infant. And, if you are breastfeeding, you should hear only positive words about your body's ability to nourish your infant and about your baby's ability to take milk. If you are feeling sad, having others listen to you without giving advice is probably what you need most. It is not always possible to delay visitors for two weeks until this fragile period is over. In the meantime, knowing that this is a normal and transient period of adjustment can help everyone.

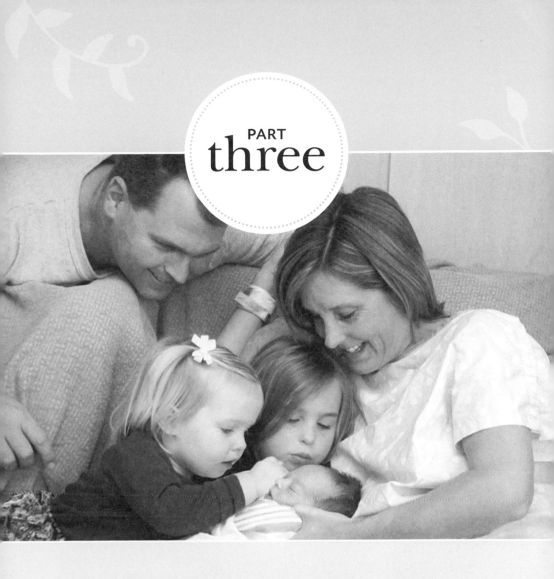

PULLING IT ALL TOGETHER

chapter 15

BIRTH YOUR WAY

THE PRECEDING PAGES GIVE MUCH detailed advice about envisioning your baby's birth and handling the different stages of labor. But on the day that you give birth you will not have time to consult hundreds of pages. You will have to pull all this advice together in your mind and in your body. Here I offer an in-depth story of how the principles of this book worked for one family. This couple succeeded in achieving empowering, natural births in two hospitals. You can see how they "pulled it all together" to create the births they wanted, especially the second time around. With love and determination, you can do the same.

Shannon and Kevin's Story

When Shannon, a mother of two, heard that I was writing a book about natural birth in hospitals, her ears perked up. "It's definitely possible to do it," she said. "Hard, but possible. You have to be ready to stand up for yourself."

Shannon's experience clearly demonstrates the difference between assertiveness and confrontation with the staff. She said that she and her husband hated the natural-birth class that they took in Berkeley, California. The teacher told the students that if they wanted to give birth in a hospital, they had to be ready to "fight." She tried to get them ready to do battle. Shannon was disappointed by this approach; she wanted an atmosphere of cooperation at her birth. When Shannon went into labor, she and her husband, Kevin, brought with them a calm sense of purpose that ultimately won most of the staff to their side.

Like many other women, Shannon wanted a hospital birth primarily for the comfort of knowing that if an emergency arose, a plethora of life-saving equipment and know-how would be in the room. Yet Shannon had a deep desire for and a deep trust in natural birth. She believed that she could give birth to her babies naturally, and she did. What Shannon learned from giving birth in a hospital the first time helped her design a second birth that came even closer to her ideal experience.

Shannon's First Birth Experience

When Shannon became pregnant the first time, her gynecologist, whom she had been seeing since puberty, told her matter-of-factly, "I'm going to deliver this baby." Shannon agreed, as much out of a feeling of obligation as anything else. She did not know until much later in her pregnancy that her doctor was the head of obstetrics at their local hospital and that he had had little experience with natural childbirth. In fact, it wasn't until her thirty-five-week appointment that she ran squarely into his real feelings about birth. At that visit, she tried to go over her birth plan with him.

"The best part of our anti-hospital childbirth class was making the birth plan," Shannon recalls. "It really got Kevin and me on the same page, working together." But when she told her obstetrician that she was planning a natural birth, he shook his head and muttered, "Whatever you want, but I don't understand you women. If I were a woman, I'd take all the drugs!" And then he added, "I don't want you to get in any funny positions. I have a bad back. I'm not going to get on the floor, you know."

Shannon did not respond because she couldn't think of what to say. "He's an older gentleman, and I didn't know what to expect. It was my first time," she says.

Instead of contracting privately for a doula, Shannon and Kevin decided to use the doulas-on-call service at their local hospital. This meant that the doula who attended the birth would be a stranger to them, someone they met only on the day Shannon went into labor.

Shannon knew that if her labor began with her waters breaking she would be "on the clock." Her doctor preferred women to give birth very quickly after their waters had broken, and he intervened aggressively to make sure that they did. Unfortunately, her labor did indeed begin with her waters breaking, at 6 a.m. She called the doula service to have a doula assigned to her. Contractions were about twenty-five minutes apart at first, the fluid was clear, and Shannon could feel her baby moving in her belly. Confident that all was well with her baby, Shannon stayed in hourly phone contact with her doula. After a few hours, the doula suggested that Shannon and Kevin, who lived about forty-five minutes away from the hospital, move closer. They went to Shannon's brother's house. She remembers walking outdoors there for hours in beautiful weather.

On the phone. her doula supported Shannon in her desire to wait until she was in active labor to go to the hospital. Contractions slowly started getting closer and closer together and more intense. Shannon started vomiting, and at some points, she would throw up after every contraction. (This isn't so unusual; many women vomit during one or more periods in labor.) Around 6 p.m., twelve hours after her waters had broken, contractions were strong and steady at three to five minutes apart. Shannon and Kevin decided to go to the hospital.

At the hospital, a nurse performed a vaginal exam and pronounced Shannon to be in active labor and 4 centimeters dilated. The nurses called Shannon's doctor, who was, in Shannon's words, "very pissed off" that she wasn't already on Pitocin to hurry her labor. "He told the nurses to get me on Pitocin immediately," Shannon remembers. But she wanted a natural birth and told the nurses so. "They were very nervous about my doctor, because he was the head of the department," recalls Shannon. They telephoned him again, and he said, "Get her on Pitocin!"

Kevin and Shannon quietly held their ground. Shannon was certain that her labor was progressing because soon after she arrived she felt herself going into what she describes as "La La Land." She and Kevin expressed their confidence to the nurses. One, Shannon remembers, was genuinely supportive. With the help of this nurse, Shannon kept on laboring naturally.

When she had reached 7 centimeters, a new nurse arrived in the room and asked without prelude, "So you're at 7 centimeters. Ready for your drugs?" Shannon was incredulous. She remembers thinking, "Isn't it in my chart what I want?" She had given a copy of her birth plan to her doctor and also submitted a copy to the hospital during a prelabor check-in.

Shannon's doula entered the room around 8 p.m. She later wrote in her notes that when she arrived, Shannon seemed "quiet and relaxed." Unfortunately, "probably because we didn't know her beforehand," the doula did not contribute much to Shannon's experience. She offered aromatherapy, but the fumes just bothered Shannon. She did help Kevin apply hot compresses and went on errands for ice chips and other things. But without the trust and intimacy that normally develop between doula and client during pregnancy, the doula seemed like "just an extra person in the room." Her positive contribution had mostly been on the phone, in helping Shannon determine when to go to the hospital.

Shannon found that showering helped ease the pain of contractions considerably. She went through transition in the shower and started to feel an urge to push around 11:30 p.m. She found herself naturally inclined to push on her hands and knees on the floor. The pushing phase lasted forty-five minutes. When her obstetrician arrived, he was irate to find her on the floor and insisted that she get on the bed. Laughing, Shannon says that "he did let me sit up and pull on a bar that they had above the bed."

The obstetrician's attitude toward natural birth had not improved since Shannon's thirty-five-week appointment. He shook his head through the delivery, muttering, "I don't know why you women want to do this." He offered her drugs, even though it was too late for an epidural. And Shannon, despite her firm commitment to natural birth, felt close to accepting them. She says that what got her through were thoughts "of the millions of women before me who have given birth without drugs, in deserts, in caves, everywhere." The doctor respected her wish to avoid an episiotomy, and she did tear some. He kept shaking his head with incredulity as he repaired her natural tear.

"Ultimately," Shannon says, "he was outnumbered." By the time the doctor had arrived on the scene, Shannon's nurses had come to understand her determination. They had witnessed her make it through active labor and transition with the full support of her husband. They had heard her quietly but firmly refuse Pitocin and continuous fetal monitoring. "I think it was my resolve that convinced them," Shannon says proudly. "I was so sure that everything was going well. I could feel things moving, I could feel the baby's head pressing down. I knew I was progressing."

Ideally, such an atmosphere of trust and confidence is created and fostered by the hospital staff for the laboring woman. But trust and confidence work in both directions. In Shannon's case, her own confidence, her husband's confidence, and the presence of a doula were enough to set the tone. The doctor muttered, but ultimately, he did not unduly intervene.

Shannon's Second Birth Experience

The second time around, Shannon and Kevin lived in the Midwest. They decided to hire hospital-based midwives in the hope of getting more active support for a natural birth. In particular, Shannon wanted to give birth on her hands and knees this time. After her first baby's birth, she was sure that this was the right delivery position for her, and she didn't want to be told to lie on her back again.

Shannon and Kevin were successful in getting most of the support that they wanted. The midwives agreed to Shannon's request about delivery position. And they did not offer drugs during labor or belittle her choices, as her obstetrician had done with the first birth. The difference between the two experiences, says Kevin, was like "night and day. The obstetrician was just so rigid, and the midwives were completely laid-back."

Like many midwives who work primarily in hospitals, however, Shannon's had rarely attended a natural birth. Most women in their care opted for epidurals and other interventions. And, like all hospital midwives in Shannon's town, Shannon's midwives worked in shifts. Shannon saw a different midwife in the practice at each prenatal visit, and until she arrived at the hospital, she did not know which would attend the birth.

Shannon was surprised that none of the midwives with whom she met would guarantee to support her fully in her natural-birth choices.

Instead, "they told me many times that all of the drugs that an obstetrician could offer were available, anything I wanted. And when we talked about possibilities like my waters breaking early, they would say, 'Well, we have to follow hospital policies about that.' No one ever said, 'Yes, we will do everything to help you have the natural birth you want.'"

The midwives campaigned against drawing up a birth plan. They didn't want their clients to "get too stuck on a plan, because every birth is different," Shannon remembers. But Shannon and Kevin again found that writing a birth plan together was an important step in their relationship. "It brought Kevin and me together," Shannon says, "so we were on the same page. He was the one who had to communicate with the doctors and everyone."

Shannon awoke one morning and felt a big contraction that "told me I'm having this baby today." So she sent her daughter, Abigail, off to her babysitter. Regular contractions began at 1 p.m. Shannon called Kevin and told him not to hurry home, but that labor had started. Luckily, he came home by 4:30, thinking that the two of them would relax during early labor by watching a movie. Shannon laughs. "Um, no time for that."

They went straight to the hospital. When they got to the door, Shannon climbed into a wheelchair backward, kneeling with her hands on the chair back. When they arrived in triage, the nurses waved them through to a labor-and-delivery room. Then the worst part of this second birth experience occurred. A play-it-by-the-book nurse took a blood sample and barraged Shannon with medical-history questions. Shannon wanted to scream at her, "I answered these questions already! Read the forms!" Asked whether Kevin could have answered the questions, Shannon says that the nurse was "right in my face." At one point, the nurse asked a question during a contraction and "was standing there waiting, like, 'Well?' And my midwife said to her, 'Can you at least let her finish the contraction?'"

Shannon labored mostly on top of the bed, leaning forward onto a large beanbag. She gave birth about an hour and a half after arriving at the hospital, and she delivered in her favored position, on her hands and knees. This felt absolutely right to her, and everyone present supported her instinctive choice. She acknowledges, laughing, that she hadn't fully thought through the first few moments after delivery. "They passed the baby through to me, but he got all tangled up in my hospital gown. Hospital gowns are just awful!"

At both births, Shannon had a sense of vindication at the end. Her babies were born healthy: alert and aware, with a rosy skin color. "They stayed with me. They made eye contact," she says happily. "Their little systems were obviously free of drugs. Their newborn scores were all 9s and 10s" (a 10 is a top score on a newborn health assessment).

What Went Right—Key Moments

Waiting until active labor was established to go to the hospital.
In Shannon's first labor, she made a pivotal decision to get support by phone from a doula rather than check into the hospital. From the way events unfolded in the hospital, we can assume that if Shannon had arrived in early labor, when her contractions were still mild and irregular, there would have been even stronger pressure to use Pitocin. If she had arrived at noon, say, after six hours of labor, she would have been interacting with nurses every thirty minutes or so for six hours before contractions became regular and strong, and her resolve to wait likely would have been less strong. Instead of walking in the sunshine, Shannon would have been in the hospital worrying about getting labor going. At 6 p.m. Shannon was able to convince her nurses not to give her Pitocin in large part because she was clearly in active labor.

The story of Shannon's second labor illustrates the disadvantage of postponing the trip to the hospital: having to answer triage questions when you are in active labor. Make sure that your support person knows the answers to the usual questions about your medical history and is ready to take over answering them. If the nurse insists that you, the patient, must verify the information, she is likely to agree that you can just nod your head in agreement and sign the forms . . . if your supporters are ready and able to do their part.

Refusing Pitocin.
Refusing Pitocin during her first labor was also key. That Shannon and Kevin were polite but firm and direct about what they wanted helped them achieve their goal, as did their infectious confidence.

Going to her inner resources at the toughest moments.
When her doctor offered drugs for pain relief during the pushing stage, Shannon thought about all the women who had given birth naturally before her, over thousands of years, and she told herself that she could do it, too. You may have this kind of self-affirmation in you already, but if you are like most women in North America, you may need to cultivate it during your pregnancy.

Remaining upright throughout labor and using a variety of positions to ease the pain.
Until her doctor entered the room in the final few minutes, Shannon was upright through almost her entire first labor. She walked outdoors during early labor and paced indoors during active labor, and she used the hospital shower during the toughest time, transition.

In her second labor, Shannon stayed at home until two hours before the delivery. In the hospital, she labored on her knees, leaning against a beanbag. She gave birth on her hands and knees.

Feeling confident.
Shannon's confidence in her ability to give birth naturally oozes out of her. This is a woman who believes in her body and expresses amazement at what it can do, "with no direction from me." Confidence is often the difference between a natural birth and medical intervention in the hospital. Nurses are used to women who say they want to "give natural birth a try." They are less used to women who say, "I believe that I can do it." When Shannon's nurses felt intimidated by her doctor's phone orders, Shannon and Kevin emphasized that Shannon could feel what was happening. She *knew* everything was going well.

Many first-time mothers do not feel confident enough to say this about their own labors. They may think, "Well, I've never been in labor before. How can I know what it's supposed to be like?" But Shannon had experienced twelve hours of a slowly building labor. Those were twelve hours of deep and intense experience with her own body. She did know that things were going well. She had felt the inexorable progress of labor.

The difference between these attitudes—between giving natural birth a try and being confident that you can do it—is as big as the Grand Canyon. And the effect on nurses, doctors, and midwives of witnessing a woman exude continuous confidence over the course of her labor can be profound. When that confidence is mirrored by the woman's partner and other support people, it is even more effective. Some medical professionals (such as Shannon's first obstetrician) manage to scoff at the idea of natural birth no matter what, but I have seen seasoned nurses and obstetricians ultimately join the cheering squad for a woman who is giving natural birth her absolute all.

Pulling It All Together for Your Family

During pregnancy, you have many tasks to complete to get ready for your natural birth. If you were giving birth two hundred years ago, you might not have to develop yourself in so many areas as women do now. To succeed at natural birth in modern hospitals, however, you need to prepare yourself emotionally, intellectually, physically, and socially. You will no doubt need more work in some areas than in others. Only you know what particular challenges you face:

Emotionally: You can explore your fears about giving birth and your hopes for the experience. You can inventory how you have felt about events in your past and learn from them as you plan for this big day. If you have any particular challenges, such as a history of trauma or anxiety, you can address them as best you can during pregnancy. You can come to terms with your thoughts and feelings about potential problems that could occur during pregnancy and birth.

Intellectually: You can do research about birth. This may be especially important if you have already had a baby and need more information about what happened at that child's birth. You can seek information that is practical and helpful and stories that are supportive and nurturing, not panic-inducing.

Physically: You can nurture yourself in pregnancy by eating well and getting a healthy dose of exercise. Through deliberate practice, such as yoga, you can rehearse breathing and relaxing while some muscles are engaged in hard work. You can also practice several different positions for labor.

Socially: You can build a birth team that supports your birth plan and learn how to interact with hospital personnel positively. You can plan to include friends and family members with the birth and baby in ways that honor your needs, not just in ways that keep the peace.

I wrote this book because I believe that all these areas deserve attention. Neglecting any one area can mean the difference between a successful natural birth and a failed attempt to get what you truly want. Every year, thousands of American and Canadian women desire but fail to achieve natural births in hospitals. This often results from focusing on one area of preparation but neglecting another. Some women equip themselves primarily with intellectual knowledge of birth. They can quote statistics about C-sections or episiotomies but fail to prepare for the pain of labor. They avoid deep introspection, and they avoid confronting their own emotions about birth, especially any feelings of fear. Other women go to the other extreme. They prepare for the internal challenges of giving birth by writing, painting, doing yoga, or meditating, but they ignore the realities of the medical world, and these realities overtake them in labor. Finally, some women might prepare internally for birth and do the intellectual research, but they do not do the social work of team building. Instead, they arm themselves as if they were going to war with their care providers. They forget that such a stance will work against their own desire for a natural birth. Making peace with your care providers is as important as finding your own position in labor.

I have outlined steps in this book to help you in all these areas: emotional, intellectual, physical, and social. If one area is particularly challenging for you, consider investing in a special class or another book. You will find lists of helpful books, videos, and websites in the "Reeferences" section at the end of this book.

I hope that Shannon and Kevin's story, and the other stories in this book, inspire you. These families have applied the principles of this book to create safe and satisfying birth experiences for themselves and their babies. The skills and preparation that they brought to their labors were wide-ranging. The couples in this book wrote birth plans. They developed supportive birth teams by remaining focused on their desire for a natural birth even when conditions were hostile (for instance, when Shannon's first obstetrician did not agree with her way of birthing). They arrived at the hospital when the mother was in active labor. You have met women in this book who were prepared for labor pain and had many skills available to them if they encountered a plateau or other labor challenge. They were prepared to handle well-meaning suggestions of unnecessary interventions with equanimity.

Like anything worthwhile, natural birth is hard work. But if you work consciously in all the areas that this book outlines, you will give yourself and your baby the best chance to start this new life with confidence, courage, and grace. When you have given birth naturally, you will move forward in your life with the knowledge that nature works in you. Women who have given birth naturally find that the gift of this knowledge follows them everywhere—into parenting, into their careers, and into their personal relationships.

I wish for you a peaceful beginning to parenthood. After all your careful preparation, I hope that you will feel more capable than ever before. The Hollywood treatment of birth is sentimental, certainly, but it also paints birth as scary, difficult, messy, and unappealing. Women who have had beautiful birth experiences describe them very differently. They use words like *amazing, empowering,* and *incredible.* By allowing hospital doctors, midwives, and nurses to witness our profound physical, mental, and emotional capacities in giving birth naturally, we can create a new image of birth.

The wonder of bringing new life into this world deserves our awe. I thank you for the hard work that you are doing. As mothers, we are literally building humanity, and I passionately believe that how we do so matters. Your baby's birth happens privately, yet it has the potential to positively affect our wider world. By respecting nature in pregnancy and birth, we are paving the way to a society more respectful of nature both in and around us.

Appendix

COMMON MEDICAL INTERVENTIONS AND HOW TO AVOID THEM

THIS LIST IS ARRANGED in the order in which you would normally encounter interventions.

Induction by Chemicals

What It Is

A medical induction is usually a two-part process. Some hospitals send you home for the first part, and some admit you for the entire procedure. The first part consists of inserting a prostaglandin gel (such as Cervidil) in the vagina to get the cervix ready for labor. The second part is administering Pitocin by IV. Some practitioners use the drug misoprostol, also called Cytotec.

Points to Consider

Of all the interventions, you may have the most control over this one. Though you might feel great pressure at the end of your pregnancy to have labor induced, research your decision carefully. Almost 40 percent of American women have inductions. Yet about a third of all inductions do not work. Once you are admitted to the hospital, everyone expects a baby to be born soon, so a "failed" induction can lead to a cesarean section. Women whose labors are induced are more likely to have C-sections than women who begin labor naturally.

An induced labor requires you to stay in bed, tethered to monitors and a blood-pressure cuff. You will probably have continuous electronic fetal monitoring (see "Electronic Fetal Monitoring," page 258, to learn what effects this can have on your birth experience). Internal fetal monitoring (using an electrode that is literally screwed into the baby's scalp) is used more often with inductions than with natural labors.

The contractions caused by Pitocin are described by women as harder and more painful than natural contractions, with multiple peaks of pain. The combination of more painful contractions and limited mobility often leads women to request pharmaceutical pain relief.

Misoprostol (also called Cytotec) has never been studied for safe use in pregnancy. Many serious side effects have been noted when it is used, off-label, in labor. In the past, mostly obstetricians used Cytotec and midwives avoided it. In the last few years, there has been increased acceptance among midwives of Cytotec for induction. Practitioners are using smaller doses than in the past, which appears to reduce some of the serious side effects. Still, the evidence is not yet robust or convincing that Cytotec is safe. Considering that the known side effects of the larger dosage include death, uterine rupture, and hemorrhage, we need stronger evidence based on larger studies that this new approach of using 25 micrograms instead of 50 is really a safe method of induction.

As of 2017, the FDA had not approved misoprostol for use in pregnancy or labor, stating on its website that "no company has sent the FDA scientific proof that misoprostol is safe and effective for these uses."

Medical studies suggest that induction should be saved for serious complications.

How to Avoid This Intervention

- Do research on your particular situation. There are only a few serious medical reasons that you would need an induction. (Going past your due date is not a serious medical reason.)

- Talk to your doula, if you have one, for emotional support in making the right decision for yourself.

- Try natural means of getting labor started, such as long walks, nipple stimulation, sexual intercourse, acupressure points, herbs such as black or blue cohosh, homeopathic remedies, or, as a last resort, castor oil. For more information, see page 117.

- Ask your care provider to try "stripping" your membranes—that is, using a finger inserted through the cervix to separate the membranes from the lower part of the uterus. This is an intervention, certainly, but it usually does not lead into the cascade of other interventions the way that Cervidil, Pitocin, misoprostol, or breaking the bag of waters do.

Your Birth Plan

Write in your plan: "I would like to allow labor to begin naturally." Be sure to talk to your care provider about the two most common reasons for induction: going past your due date and having your waters break before contractions begin.

Induction by Breaking the Bag of Waters

What It Is

Your care provider inserts an object that resembles a long crochet hook into your vagina and nicks the bag of waters to open it.

Points to Consider

Since the bag of waters protects the baby and your uterus from coming into contact with germs, when the bag is broken, your care provider will be concerned that you or your baby could develop an infection. An infection inside your uterus is potentially very serious. After the membranes are broken, most care providers operate with a time limit on labor, from about twelve hours to about twenty-four hours. If by the end of that time you have not given birth and are not in active, progressing labor, your care provider will likely suggest interventions such as Pitocin to make contractions stronger or a cesarean section.

Another risk to induction by breaking your bag of waters is that, if you develop a fever, your care provider will probably want your baby to be born as soon as possible because there is no way to know whether the fever indicates an infection in the uterus.

How to Avoid This Intervention

• Avoid induction by chemical means. When pharmaceutical induction doesn't work, the next step is often breaking the bag of waters.

- Say, "We'd like to wait an hour" when this intervention is suggested.

- Attempt to get labor started by natural means (see pages 116 and 117).

Your Birth Plan
Write in your birth plan: "I would like to allow labor to begin naturally."

Induction by Foley Bulb
What It Is
Foley bulbs are usually used after chemicals such as Cytotec or Cervidil have ripened your cervix. Rubber tubing is inserted through your vagina and stuck into the cervical opening. Then the tubing is inflated, which puts mechanical pressure on your cervix to open. When your cervix opens to 3 cm, the Foley bulb falls out. Most women find the process of inserting the Foley bulb quite painful. Some, but not all, women find that pain continues the whole time that the Foley bulb is pushing on the cervix. Foley bulbs are usually inserted for three to twelve hours. Some hospitals will send women home in the evening with a Foley bulb inserted and advise that they return the next morning (or earlier, if contractions begin). The hope is that mechanical opening of a woman's cervix will throw her into labor.

How to Avoid This Intervention
Overall, avoiding induction completely is usually your best option. In the case of a true medical need for induction, induction by Foley bulb is less invasive of your overall system than many other methods. There are no chemicals or hormones; it is purely mechanical. If you are choosing induction, this method is probably more conducive to having a natural labor afterward than is induction by Pitocin.

Your Birth Plan
Planning to avoid induction altogether is your best plan. Write in your plan: "I would like to allow labor to begin naturally." Be sure to talk to your care provider about the two most common reasons for induction: going past your due date and having your waters break before contractions begin. However, if you fall into the small percentage of women who

have a true medical need for an induction, consider the Foley bulb method before Pitocin.

Vaginal Examinations

What They Are

In most hospitals, vaginal examinations are performed routinely. Depending on how far along you are in labor, you can expect a vaginal examination every two hours, every hour, or every half hour. During the pushing stage, some practitioners make very frequent checks or even keep their hands inside a woman's vagina almost continuously to feel the baby's movement downward.

Points to Consider

Most of the time, care providers will ask women to get onto the bed for a vaginal check. The position is often painful for laboring women. And the vaginal examination itself can be quite painful, especially during a contraction.

If your waters have broken, vaginal examinations can increase your chance of infection. In this case, most natural-birth advocates suggest that you avoid routine vaginal exams.

During early and active labor, you may or may not want to have vaginal exams. Sometimes, hearing how far your cervix has dilated might help your confidence. But you might feel discouraged to hear that you are not as far along as you had hoped.

In late labor, and especially if you have been pushing for a long time, your caregiver may want to do a vaginal check not to check for cervical dilation but to feel for the baby's position. By touching the bones of the baby's head, your caregiver can determine whether the baby is in a favorable position.

Women who have experienced sexual abuse in their past may have a strong negative reaction to vaginal examinations.

How to Avoid This Intervention

Think ahead of time about whether you are likely to want vaginal examinations to check your cervical progress. If you want to refuse or minimize vaginal exams, make sure that your support team knows how you feel.

If you are undecided, remember that during labor you can always say, "I'd like to wait an hour," to give yourself more time to think. You might avoid a check in early labor, when the result might be discouraging, but welcome a check during transition, when you might need to hear that you are nearly 10 centimeters dilated.

Be prepared to be firm, but polite. Whereas your care provider is likely to believe that some interventions are absolutely essential, she is unlikely to believe that vaginal examinations are necessary for your health. Refusing vaginal examinations throughout labor requires steadfastness, but I have seen women succeed.

Your Birth Plan

Because this is an issue negotiated in labor, usually with nurses rather than the care provider, it generally should be handled in person and left out of the birth plan you bring to the hospital.

Electronic Fetal Monitoring

Points to Consider

Monitoring your baby's heart rate during labor is a good idea, but you do not have to use an electronic fetal monitor (EFM) to do so.

When you are connected to an EFM machine, you lose mobility. During active labor, this can impair your ability to cope with contractions. Lying in bed, you are also more likely to feel helpless more so than you would if you were active and on your feet.

The baby's heart rate normally changes during labor. When you are connected to a machine, every little change is recorded. Many studies have indicated that caregivers are more likely to intervene, including with C-section, because of electronic fetal monitoring. Even in cases when serious interventions are avoided, the family can experience unnecessary scares that something is wrong with the baby. This experience of fear can negatively affect your labor.

Because the EFM machine also reports the intensity of contractions, many women find that their partners and nurses pay more attention to the machine than to them.

Often, nurses will request a "twenty-minute strip" on an EFM machine. After you are connected to the machine, however, the nurse is likely to leave the room. She may not return for forty minutes or more. In the meantime, if you take off the monitor or the blood-pressure cuff, the machines start to beep and blare.

How to Avoid This Intervention

Ask your caregiver to use a handheld Doppler, an ultrasound stethoscope. Some midwives might even agree to monitor your baby's heartbeat with a fetoscope, a fetal stethoscope that does not use ultrasound. Either of these alternatives allows you to remain upright and mobile (and possibly even to take a bath or shower). Besides, if your nurses use a handheld device, they can't leave the room with you tethered to machines.

Your Birth Plan

Write in your birth plan: "Please use a handheld Doppler or fetoscope to monitor the baby's heart rate."

Epidural

Points to Consider

The upside of an epidural is that you potentially feel no pain during labor. In some cases, women still feel pain or pressure on one or both sides of their body even with an epidural.

The downside of an epidural includes many potential complications. There are the serious complications that the anesthesiologist might breeze through on the consent form, such as temporary or permanent paralysis (rare, yet common enough that I have personally seen two cases of temporary paralysis) and intense headaches that can last for days or even weeks (these are relatively common). Taking care of a newborn in the middle of the night with an epidural headache is horrible.

Other complications are not on the consent form, but can be serious:

• In most hospitals, with an epidural you are committed to lying on your back for the rest of the birth (the term *walking epidural* usually means that the medicine level is low, but does not mean that you can actually walk or even stand). If your baby's heart rate slows because the umbilical cord is compressed, you will not be able to change position much.

- You will not be able to walk or change position if labor plateaus.

- Nor will you be able to easily change position if your baby's shoulders get stuck in the birth canal. Changing position is the age-old solution to this complication, which can be life-threatening for your baby. With an epidural, however, a more invasive solution, such as cutting a large episiotomy or breaking the baby's shoulder bone, is usually employed.

- If you cannot feel enough to push effectively, your baby might need to be delivered by forceps or vacuum. Each of these carries its own risks for the baby.

How to Avoid This Intervention
- Allow labor to begin spontaneously.

- Hire a doula.

- Go to the hospital only after labor is well established.

- Practice different positions, words of encouragement, visualizations, and meditation techniques during pregnancy.

- Appoint another person to answer questions at the hospital.

Your Birth Plan
Write: "Please help me achieve the most natural birth possible" and "Please do not offer any pain medication during labor, even if I look like I am in pain."

Episiotomy

What It Is
An episiotomy is a cut in the perineum, the area between your vagina and anus, made with scissors.

Points to Consider
In rare cases, this surgical enlargement of the vagina is necessary and helpful (for instance, if your baby must be delivered by forceps). Most of the time, however, episiotomies are not medically necessary. In addition,

they take longer to heal than natural tears. Tears are usually small and superficial, although they may occur in several places. Repairing tears with sutures may take more of a caregiver's time than stitching up a deep cut, but natural tears are usually less painful in the weeks after the birth.

How to Avoid This Intervention

- Choose a caregiver who seldom performs episiotomies and doesn't believe in doing so routinely.

- Do Kegel exercises (see page 224) during your third trimester.

- Do vaginal massage with oil during your third trimester to stretch your tissues. Use any vegetable oil, such as olive or almond, or a water-soluble lubricant such as K-Y.

- Ask for hot compresses to be placed against your perineum during the pushing phase, especially toward the end.

- Push slowly—or, better yet, don't push at all!—as your baby crowns at birth. Give your body time to stretch.

Your Birth Plan

You might write: "I prefer to use hot compresses and possibly tear naturally during birth rather than have an episiotomy."

Routine Pitocin After the Placenta Is Delivered

What It Is

Virtually all hospitals now routinely administer a pharmaceutical drug such as Pitocin after the placenta is delivered to help the uterus clamp down and stop bleeding.

Points to Consider

If you have just given birth naturally, you probably do not embrace the idea of the routine use of a pharmaceutical agent to help your uterus function. If you have previously experienced a hemorrhage, you know that you have low iron, or you have a long labor (meaning, your uterine muscles are more tired), you may be a good candidate for this intervention.

How to Avoid This Intervention

To make sure that you will be at low risk for a postpartum hemorrhage, you can try the following:

- Avoid induction or augmentation with synthetic oxytocin (such as Pitocin) during your labor.

- Eat and drink during labor.

- Make sure that you are not anemic in your last trimester. Women who are anemic have worse consequences from small amounts of blood loss than do women who have iron-rich blood. Eat a lot of iron-rich foods and take a supplement, if necessary. Many women find the natural formula of Floradix, a liquid iron supplement found at many health food stores, easier on their digestive systems than iron pills.

- Be aware that long labors (more than 24 hours) may mean that your uterine muscles are more tired than they would be otherwise. Think ahead of time about whether you would feel differently about this intervention if your labor goes longer than 24 hours.

Your Birth Plan

Make sure to let your support people know that you do not want routine Pitocin after you give birth. In some hospitals, I have seen Pitocin given without any notice to the mother, even though her birth plan has said she did not want it. You might write in your birth plan: "I prefer to allow my uterus to clamp down naturally after birth." Alternatively, you may write that you want to consider the length of your labor before you make a final decision. For example, since length of labor is a factor in postpartum hemorrhage, you may decide to accept this intervention if your labor is long, but refuse it if your labor is short.

References

Althabe, F., & Belizán, J. F. (2006). "Caesarean Section: The Paradox." *The Lancet (368)*: 1472–73.

Bernstein, P. (1993). *Having a Baby: Mothers Tell Their Stories.* New York, NY: Pocket Books.

Betrán, J. A., Merialdi, M., Lauer, Bing-Shun, W., Thomas, J., Van Look, P., & Wagner, M. (2007). "Rates of Caesarean Section: Analysis of Global, Regional and National Estimates." *Paediatric and Perinatal Epidemiology 21*: 98–113.

The Boston Women's Health Collective. (2008). *Our Bodies, Ourselves: Pregnancy and Birth.* New York, NY: Simon & Schuster.

Bowers, N. (2001). *The Multiple Pregnancy Sourcebook.* Naperville, IL: Sourcebooks.

Burnett, D., Phillips, G., & Tashani, O. A. (2017). "The Effect of Brief Mindfulness Meditation on Cold-Pressor Induced Pain Responses in Healthy Adults." *Pain Studies and Treatment 5*: 11–19. DOI:10.4236/pst.2017.52002

Centers for Disease Control and Prevention. (2010). "Prevention of Perinatal Group B Streptococcal Disease." *Morbidity and Mortality Weekly Report 59*(RR-10): 1–32.

Centers for Disease Control and Prevention. (2002). "Prevention of Perinatal Group B Streptococcal Disease." *Morbidity and Mortality Weekly Report 51*(RR-11): 1–22.

Cesario, S. K. (2004). "Managing the Second Stage of Labor: Using Evidence to Guide Practice." *Worldviews on Evidence-Based Nursing 1*(4): 230.

Chandraharan, E., & Arulkumaran, S. (2007). "Prevention of Birth Asphyxia: Responding Appropriately to Cardiotocograph (CTG) Traces." *Best Practice and Research Clinical Obstetrics and Gynaecology 21*(4): 609–24.

Csikszentmihalyi, M. (2008). *Flow: The Psychology of Optimal Experience.* New York, NY: Harper Perennial.

Davis, E. (2004). *Heart and Hands: A Midwife's Guide to Pregnancy and Birth.* 4th ed. New York, NY: Celestial Arts Publishing/10 Speed Press.

Davis-Floyd, R. E. (2004). *Birth as an American Rite of Passage.* Berkeley, CA: University of California Press.

Davis-Floyd, R., Barclay, L., Daviss B.-A., & Tritten, J. (2009). *Birth Models That Work.* Berkeley, CA: University of California Press.

Declercq, E. R., Sakala, C., Corry, M. P., Applebaum, S., & Herrlich, A. (2014). "Major Survey Findings of Listening to Mothers III: Pregnancy and Birth." *Journal of Perinatal Education 23*(1): 9–16.

Dekker, R. (2017). "Evidence On: Induction When Your Water Breaks at Term (PROM)." https://evidencebasedbirth.com/evidence-inducing-labor-water-breaks-term/

Duncan, L., Cohn, M., Chao, M., Cook, J., Riccobono, J., & Bardacke, N. (2017). "Benefits of Preparing for Childbirth with Mindfulness Training: A Randomized Controlled Trial with Active Comparison." *BMC Pregnancy and Childbirth 17*(140): 1–11. DOI: 10.1186/s12884-017-1319-3

Feldman, R., Rosenthal, Z., & Eidelman, A. (2014). "Maternal-Preterm Skin-To-Skin Contact Enhances Child Physiologic Organization and Cognitive Control Across the First 10 Years of Life." *Biological Psychiatry 75*(1): 56–64.

Gaskin, I. M. (2003). *Ina May's Guide to Childbirth.* New York, NY: Bantam Dell.

Goer, H. (1995). *Obstetric Myths versus Research Realities.* Westport, CT: Bergin and Garvey.

———. (1999). *The Thinking Woman's Guide to a Better Birth.* New York, NY: Berkeley Publishing Group.

Goetzl, L., Rivers, J., Evans, T., Citron, D. R., Richardson, B. E., Lieberman, E., & Suresh, M. S. (2004). "Prophylactic Acetaminophen Does Not Prevent Epidural Fever in Nulliparous Women: A Double-Blind Placebo-Controlled Trial." *Journal of Perinatology 24*: 471–75.

Gottschalk, A., & Flocke, S. A. (2005). "Time Spent in Face-to-Face Patient Care and Work Outside the Examination Room." *Annals of Family Medicine 3*: 488–93.

Gupta, J., Sood, A., Hofmeyr, G. J., & Vogel, J. (2017). "Position in the Second Stage of Labour for Women without Epidural Anaethesia." *Cochrane Database of Systemic Reviews 5.* DOI: 10.1002/14651858.CD002006.pub4

Hannah, M. E. (1996). "Induction of Labor Compared with Expectant Management for Prelabor Rupture of the Membranes at Term." *New England Journal of Medicine 334*(16): 1005–10.

Harper, B. (2005). *Gentle Birth Choices*. Rochester, NY: Healing Arts Press.

Hiersch, L., Krispin, E., Aviram, A., Mor-Shacham, M., Gabbay-Benziv, R., Yogev, Y., & Ashwal, E. (2017). "Predictors for Prolonged Interval from Premature Rupture of Membranes to Spontaneous Onset of Labor at Term." *Journal of Maternal-Fetal & Neonatal Medicine 30*(12): 1465–1470.

Huggins, K. (2017). *The Nursing Mother's Companion*. 7th ed. Beverly, MA: Harvard Common Press.

Johnson, K. C., & Daviss, B.-A. (2005). "Outcomes of Planned Home Births with Certified Professional Midwives: Large Prospective Study in North America." *British Medical Journal 330*: 1416.

Klaus, M. H., Kennell, J. H., & Klaus, P. H. (2002). *The Doula Book: How a Trained Labor Companion Can Help You Have a Shorter, Easier, and Healthier Birth*. New York, NY: Da Capo Press.

Lauderdale, D. S. (2006). "Birth Outcomes for Arabic-Named Women in California before and after September 11." *Demography 43*(1): 185–201.

Layard, R. (2005). *Happiness: Lessons from a New Science*. New York, NY: Penguin Group.

Lengelle, R. (2005). "Reinekke Lengelle's Birth Story." In J. Schwegel (Ed.), *Adventures in Natural Childbirth: Tales from Women on the Joys, Fears, Pleasures, and Pains of Giving Birth Naturally* (pp. 55–58). New York, NY: Marlowe and Company.

Lenihan, J. P. (1984). "Relationship of antepartum pelvic examinations to premature rupture of the membranes." *Obstetrics and Gynecology 63*(1): 33–37.

Lieberman, E., Lang, J. M., Frigoletto Jr., F., Richardson, D. K., Ringer, S. A., & Cohen, A. (1997). "Epidural Analgesia, Intrapartum Fever, and Neonatal Sepsis Evaluation." *Pediatrics 99*(3): 415–19.

Marowitz, A., & Jordan, R. (2007). "Midwifery Management of Prelabor Rupture of Membranes at Term." *Journal of Midwifery and Women's Health 52*(3): 199–206.

Mozurkewich, E. (2006). "Prelabor Rupture of Membranes at Term: Induction Techniques." *Clinical Obstetrics and Gynecology 49*(3): 672–83.

O'Mara, P. (2003). *Mothering Magazine's Having a Baby, Naturally: The Mothering Magazine Guide to Pregnancy and Childbirth*. New York, NY: Atria Books.

Pintucci, A., Meregalli, V., Colombo, P., & Fiorilli, A. (2014). "Premature Rupture of Membranes at Term in Low Risk Women: How Long Should We Wait in the 'Latent Phase'?" *Journal of Perinatal Medicine 42*(2): 189–196.

Righard, L. (1992). *Delivery Self Attachment*. Sunland, CA: Geddes Productions.

Rooks, J. P., Weatherby, N. L., Ernst, E. K., Stapleton, S., Rosen, D., & Rosenfield, A. (1989). "Outcomes of Care in Birth Centers: The National Birth Center Study." *New England Journal of Medicine 321*: 1804–11.

Sampselle, C. M. (1992). *Violence against Women: Nursing Research, Education, and Practical Issues*. New York, NY: Hemisphere Publishing Corporation.

Shalev, E., Peleg, D., Eliyahu, S., & Nahum, Z. (1995). "Comparison of 12- and 72-Hour Expectant Management of Premature Rupture of Membranes in Term Pregnancies." *Obstetrics and Gynecology 85*(5) Part 1: 766–68.

Sharpe, E. & Arendt, K. (2017). "Epidural Labor Analgesia and Maternal Fever." *Clinical Obstetrics and Gynecology 60*(2): 365–374.

Simpson, K. R., & James, D. C. (2005). "Effects of Immediate versus Delayed Pushing during Second-Stage Labor on Fetal Well-being: A Randomized Clinical Trial." *Nursing Research 54*(3): 149–57.

Soper, D., Mayhall, C., & Froggatt, J. (1996). "Characterization and Control of Intraamniotic Infection in an Urban Teaching Hospital." *American Journal of Obstetrics and Gynecology 175*: 304–10.

Sperlich, M., & Seng, J. S. (2008). *Survivor Moms: Women's Stories of Birthing, Mothering and Healing after Sexual Abuse*. Eugene, Oregon: Motherbaby Press.

Stoll, K., & Hall, W. (2013). "Vicarious Birth Experiences and Childbirth Fear: Does It Matter How Young Canadian Women Learn About Birth?" *Journal of Perinatal Education 22*(4): 226–233.

Walls, M., Wright, A., Fowlie, P., & Hume, R. (2004). "Home Phototherapy: A Feasible, Safe and Acceptable Practice." *Journal of Neonatal Nursing 10*(3): 92–94.

Walrath, D. (2003). "Rethinking Pelvic Typologies and the Human Birth Mechanism." *Current Anthropology 44*(1): 5–31.

World Health Organization. (April 2015). "WHO Statement on Caesarean Section Rates."

Visualization and Meditation Books and CDs

Elliott, J. (2004). *Birth with Calm and Confidence.* Toronto: Life's Journey. Audio CD or MP3 download at: lifesjourney.ca/hypnosis-recordings/#birth

Garth, M. (1991). *Starbright: Meditations for Children.* New York, NY: HarperOne.

———. (1997). *Earthlight: New Meditations for Children.* New York, NY: HarperCollins.

Naparstek, B. (1999). *A Guided Meditation for Healing Trauma (PTSD).* Akron, OH: Health Journeys. Audio CD.

Group B Strep Books

Balaskas, J. (1992). *Active Birth: The New Approach to Giving Birth Naturally.* Revised ed. Boston, MA: Harvard Common Press.

Dick-Read, G. (2004). *Childbirth without Fear: The Principles and Practice of Natural Childbirth.* London, England: Pinter & Martin Ltd.

England, P. (1998). *Birthing from Within.* Albuquerque, NM: Partera Press.

Goer, H. (1999). *The Thinking Woman's Guide to a Better Birth.* New York, NY: Berkley Publishing Group.

Gurevich, R. (2003). *The Doula Advantage: Your Complete Guide to Having an Empowered and Positive Birth with the Help of a Professional Childbirth Assistant.* Roseville, CA: Prima Lifestyles.

Kitzinger, S. (2004). *The New Experience of Childbirth.* London, England: Dorling Kindersley.

Lieberman, A. B. (1992). *Easing Labor Pain: The Complete Guide to a More Comfortable and Rewarding Birth.* Boston, MA: Harvard Common Press.

Morton, C., & Clift, E. (2014). *Birth Ambassadors: Doulas and the Re-Emergence of Woman-Supported Birth in America.* Amarillo, TX: Praeclarus Press.

Mongan, M. (2005). *HypnoBirthing: The Mongan Method.* Deerfield Beach, FL: Health Communication, Inc.

Naparstek, B. (2004). *Invisible Heroes: Survivors of Trauma and How They Heal.* New York, NY: Bantam Books.

Simkin, P. (2017). *The Birth Partner: A Complete Guide to Childbirth for Dads, Doulas, and All Other Labor Companions.* 4th ed. Beverly, MA: Harvard Common Press.

Sperlich, M., & Seng, J. S. (2008). *Survivor Moms: Women's Stories of Birthing, Mothering and Healing after Sexual Abuse.* Eugene, OR: Motherbaby Press.

About the Author

Cynthia Gabriel, Ph.D., is mother to three, a birth and postpartum doula, childbirth educator, and medical anthropologist. She is the author of *The Fourth Trimester Companion*. She researches childbirth and parenting cross-culturally in Russia, Canada, the United States, and Brazil. Recent research interests include racial inequalities in childbirth; trauma survivors who give birth; and the cesarean rate in Brazil. She lives and teaches in Ann Arbor, Michigan.

Index